BEYOND
ALZHEIMER'S

C1

BEYOND ALZHEIMER'S

How to Avoid the Modern Epidemic of Dementia

Scott D. Mendelson, M.D., Ph.D.

M. EVANS
Lanham • New York • Boulder • Toronto • Plymouth, UK

Published by M. Evans
An imprint of The Rowman & Littlefield Publishing Group, Inc.
4501 Forbes Boulevard, Suite 200, Lanham, Maryland 20706
http://www.rlpgtrade.com

Estover Road, Plymouth PL6 7PY, United Kingdom

Distributed by National Book Network

British Library Cataloguing in Publication Information Available

Library of Congress Cataloging-in-Publication Data

Mendelson, Scott D.
  Beyond Alzheimer's: How to avoid the modern epidemic of dementia / Scott D. Mendelson.
    p. cm.
  ISBN 978-1-59077-157-0 (cloth : alk. paper) — ISBN 978-1-59077-158-7 (electronic)
  1. Alzheimer's disease—Prevention—Popular works. 2. Brain—Aging—Popular works. 3. Senile dementia—Nutritional aspects—Popular works. I. Title.
  RC523.2.M46 2009
  616.8'31—dc22

                                                        2009007928

Printed in the United States of America

I dedicate this book to the memory of my father, Harry Mendelson. His pleasures were the simple ones. He had a wonderful sense of humor, he loved a hearty meal on the table, and he possessed the uncanny ability to sniff out the perfect fishing hole. He was a decent, hardworking family man.

He did not deserve the fate he suffered.

CONTENTS

INTRODUCTION

The Dementia Epidemic

The incidence of Alzheimer's and other forms of dementia is increasing worldwide, and many experts have begun to warn that an epidemic is approaching. Dementia is a decline in the ability to think, remember, and use the mind to go about one's normal daily activities. It is estimated that dementia affects about twenty-five million people in the world today. This number is expected to double by 2020 and double again by 2040. The financial costs of caring for people with dementia are enormous. In the United States, annual Medicare payments for the care of patients with dementia were over $91 billion in 2005, and these are projected to increase to $160 billion by 2010. The stress and strain placed on families and caregivers costs society an extra $36 billion a year due to absenteeism and drops in productivity. The human costs are incalculable. We are only beginning to understand the tremendous emotional burden borne by spouses, daughters, and sons who provide care for those afflicted by dementia.

There are many reasons why an epidemic of dementia may be starting at this particular time in history. The most obvious reason is that our population is getting older. About 96 percent of cases of dementia occur in people over the age of sixty-five. Because of improvements in food production and health care, as well as demographic changes such as the post–World War II baby boom, there has been a dramatic increase in the number of people sixty-five years of age and older in the world. To some extent, the increase in the number of people diagnosed with dementia parallels this "graying" of the world's population.

Although part of the increase in rates of dementia can be attributed to demographic factors, there is evidence that much of it is due to unhealthy changes in our modern lifestyles. A variety of studies have shown that the risk of developing dementia increases when people from simpler cultures move to developed countries and leave their traditional lifestyles behind. For example, a recent study that compared the rates of dementia in African Americans living in the United States with those of a similar population living in their native Nigeria showed that rates were nearly doubled for those living in the United States. In another study, Japanese Americans who kept their language, diet, and other cultural habits were found to be far less likely to develop dementia than those who abandoned them after coming to the United States.

An overall decline in our health in modern times is a major factor in the increasing risk of developing dementia. The risk of dementia grows when an individual suffers diabetes, heart disease, obesity, and other major health problems. The numbers of people being diagnosed with such conditions are exploding; as with the incidence of dementia, the incidence of these illnesses is reaching epidemic proportions. There are other dangers of modern life that we can have difficulty avoiding or even recognizing. The air we breathe, the water we drink, and the food we eat frequently carry contaminants that injure our health and increase our risk of developing dementia. Modern technology, such as cell phones and other electronic devices, may make its own contribution to increasing this risk.

When memory and judgment fade in our loved ones, or in ourselves, it is common and reasonable to consider the possibility of Alzheimer's dementia. However, the cases of dementia that are being diagnosed with increasing frequency in society today have little to do with the illness first described by Dr. Alois Alzheimer in 1907. The classical form of what we call Alzheimer's dementia is the result of genetic abnormalities that cause early and rapidly progressing loss of cognitive function. While modern cases of dementia *can* be the result of genetic abnormalities, in most cases, abnormal genes are neither necessary nor sufficient to produce the degeneration of brain tissue that results in the forms of dementia commonly seen today. The damage underlying most current cases of dementia is largely the result of abnormalities we introduce into our brain chemistries as the result of unhealthy diet, poor lifestyle choices, stress, and exposure to environmental contaminants.

Some losses in cognitive function that occur with age are unavoidable. Some people are genetically predisposed to dementia of one type or another. As is the case with many maladies that plague mankind, some unfortunate individuals may be destined to suffer these illnesses of the mind and brain. However, there is compelling evidence that by improving our diet, reducing stress, exercising our minds and bodies, staying socially active, and finding emotional peace, most of us can avoid or at least delay the development of dementia.

In the following pages I will discuss normal patterns of aging and how these differ from what is seen in dementia. I will explain how a physician recognizes and diagnoses dementia and describe the different types of dementias and how they can be distinguished from one another. These discussions will be followed by an explanation of what causes dementia, including the fact that while some forms of dementia are largely genetic, most cases of dementia arise out of poor diet and other unhealthy lifestyle choices. Then I will provide the most scientifically up-to-date information about strategies for changes in diet, exercise, stress management, sleep, intellectual activity, and social interaction to help avoid these diseases of the brain. As part of my presentation, I will give detailed, scientifically sound information about a variety of herbs, vitamins, and nutraceuticals that can be taken as supplements to both improve cognitive function and help prevent or at least delay the onset of dementia.

② WHAT IS AGING?

Why do we grow old and die? At first it would seem to be the simplest of questions. The answer that first leaps to mind is that due to the wear and tear of life, the body simply gives out over time. Although this seems to be a perfectly logical explanation, it collapses under scrutiny. Cats and dogs, which exert themselves more or less the same as we humans do (my own pets considerably *less* than I do), live only twelve to fifteen years before they die. On the other hand, tortoises, which labor all their lives under a heavy shell in the most severe of environments, can often live to be well over one hundred years old. In captivity, the grim turkey buzzard has been known to live more than 110 years. The lighthearted canary may live a mere twenty. The wear-and-tear theory doesn't hold water.

Some scientists have had the audacity to question why it is that we age and die at all. In his famous 1957 paper, "Pleiotropy, Natural Selection, and the Evolution of Senescence," the biologist George C. Williams observed, "It is indeed remarkable that after a seemingly miraculous feat of morphogenesis, a complex metazoan should be unable to perform the much simpler task of merely maintaining what is already formed." In other words, after an animal has already performed the nearly impossible task of growing from a single cell to become a fully formed, mature adult, it seems that simply keeping itself alive and in good repair would hardly be a trick at all.

August Weismann, a nineteenth-century biologist, was among the first to suggest that growing old and dying was an evolutionary development that allowed older, weaker animals to leave room for younger, stronger members of the species. Disease, predators, and bad luck would eventually take their toll on individuals and weaken them over time. However, death was a more certain way to cull the herd of the damaged members, and it became a useful process to maintain the overall health of the species. Many biologists now believe life span and death are too important to be left to chance and that they are programmed into the genes of every species. It is important for there to be genes to make the young strong, competitive, and successful in reproduction. However, since death has some advantages for the species, it is likely that genetic programs evolved to make certain that every organism dies at the proper time.

Normal human cells, when grown in a petri dish, can divide a certain number of times before they stop dividing and eventually die. This phenomenon of a limited number of divisions was first noted by Leonard Hayflick in 1961, and it is known as the Hayflick limit. One factor that determines the number of times a cell can divide in culture is the length of the telomeres on the ends of each chromosome in a cell. Telomere literally means "end part," and they are special chains of DNA that cap the end of chromosomes. At first it was thought that telomeres on the ends of DNA strands simply prevented the ends from sticking to each other and tangling themselves into knots. In 1990, it was discovered that telomeres grow shorter as cells age and that the length of the telomeres is the strongest indication of how many more times a cell will be able to divide. Every time a cell divides, a small piece of telomere chain is clipped off, and, like an hourglass slowly emptying, when the last telomere is clipped off, time runs out for further cell division. Running out of telomeres does not kill the cell, but with no more new cells being produced, the organism can no longer replenish or properly repair its tissues, and it is only a matter of time before the organism wears out. Young sufferers of the tragic illness progeria have unusually short telomeres on their chromosomes, which is likely to contribute to their rapid aging and untimely death.

There is evidence that short telomeres may serve as a biological marker for increased risk of development of a condition with the self-descriptive name of mild cognitive impairment, or MCI. In many cases, MCI can progress to become dementia. Thus, the length of our telomeres, a characteristic we inherit from our parents, may help determine the length of our life span, as well as our risk for developing dementia. However, the relationship between telomere length in a cell's DNA and its ability to divide is not as absolute as it was once thought to be, and there are indications that what occurs in a petri dish is not exactly the same as what occurs in a living organism. Recent studies have found that lifestyle choices, particularly diets low in saturated fat and simple carbohydrates, can slow or even reverse the telomeric countdown. On the other hand, lengthy telomeres alone do not guarantee that cells will continue to divide and grow. Whereas it was once thought that neurons in the adult mammalian brain do not divide and replace themselves, it has been found over the past fifteen years that new neurons are born in the human brain in a process called neurogenesis. Even when telomeres are of adequate length, abnormal processes, such as persistent stress and major depression, can interfere with neurogenesis.

Telomeres don't exist simply to limit our life span.[1] It turns out that an important function of telomeres is to prevent the endless division of cells that characterizes the most dire of all struggles of life and death that can take place within an individual—that is, cancer. To protect ourselves from early death by cancer, we trade off the ability of normal cells to forever replace themselves with healthy new cells. Such trade-offs in biology are common, and George Williams explained them in his notion of "antagonistic pleiotropy," in which he theorized that some genes have evolved to have more than one effect on cells and organisms. Whereas one effect of the gene may increase survival in certain situations, others of its effects can be detrimental. Simply stated, to grow, thrive, reproduce, and compete, organisms mortgage their futures by investing in cellular chemistries that give them advantages early in life, but later leave them impoverished and dying.

Genetic programs for life and death exist not only for the individual, but also for cells within the individual. Scientists have discovered that while some cells within an organism may die from infection or injury, others die in an orderly fashion called apoptosis.[2] Some scientists refer to this as "programmed cellular suicide." If a cell is no longer functioning properly, if it contains viruses, or if it has fallen victim to inflammatory processes in the body, it responds to chemical signals to turn itself off. Sometimes these signals are sent by neighboring cells, and sometimes the signal arises from deep inside its own cellular structures. There are also circumstances in

---

1. Contrary to expectations, there is not a clear relationship between the length of the telomeres of any specific species of animal and its longevity relative to other species. For example, mice live much shorter lives than humans, but their telomeres are substantially longer. This simply shows that there are factors other than length of telomeres that determine longevity. Nonetheless, a mouse with long telomeres might yet be expected to live longer than a mouse with much shorter telomeres.

2. Exactly how to pronounce the word "apoptosis" is one of the great controversies of modern science. When fistfights break out at the annual conference of the Society for Neuroscience, you can safely assume that it is due either to a bad debt, a romantic triangle of some sort, or a heated argument over the pronunciation of apoptosis. Some say ā pŏp tō sĭs. However, since the word is derived from Greek, I believe the preferred pronunciation is with the second "p" silent, in other words, ā pō tō sĭs.

which a brain cell can be stimulated, or perhaps the more accurate word is "tricked," into prematurely and unnecessarily initiating its apoptosis program. These circumstances can arise under conditions of stress, poor sleep, poor diet, and metabolic syndrome, which I will later describe in detail.

Although DNA holds the instructions for how each cell in the body operates, there are many physiological and environmental factors that can affect which genes are allowed to have their say. For example, restriction of food intake can increase the life span of animals as varied as yeast, worms, and flies. It has recently been shown that this can also increase the longevity of mammals. These effects are mediated by activation of sirtuins. The sirtuins are a class of proteins that help repair DNA, as well as control which genes in the chain of DNA are expressed. Sirtuins increase life span in part by inhibiting apoptosis. Sirtuins may also protect the brain and defend against dementia by keeping neurons alive during times of stress and injury. Unfortunately, there is a trade-off, or what might be seen as yet another example of antagonistic pleiotropy. Sirtuins divert neural progenitor cells, infant cells otherwise earmarked for development into neurons through the process of neurogenesis, to instead develop into a type of custodial cells known as astrocytes. Astrocytes help protect and defend neurons, but their birth may come at the expense of the brain not replacing neurons that do perish.

Death is programmed into the genes of every animal. Yet, why is it that some species of animals live longer than others? Why, for example, do we live longer than our pets? Predatory animals, such as lions and wolves, and their cousins, our pet cats and dogs, have little to offer other members of their species when they have grown too old to hunt for food. After they reproduce, it is most beneficial for the group for the older animals to die to allow more food for the younger, stronger animals. We humans, however, are different in an important respect. We are gifted by nature with remarkable brains and the capacity not only to learn, but to pass on this knowledge to our children and grandchildren through language. The elderly possess knowledge and wisdom that can greatly benefit the young, and it is to our species' advantage for some members to continue to live beyond their years of reproduction and peak physical strength to pass on that knowledge. It is reasonable to assume that our DNA programs us not only to live well beyond our reproductive years, but also to retain our unique mental faculties over the length of our lives to allow us to convey this knowledge to our young.[3]

---

3. It is fair to argue that the tortoise rarely has much of consequence to communicate to its offspring, and that living long to pass on knowledge cannot explain the longevity of this and certain other species of animal. I agree. However, teaching the young, such as occurs in humans, great

Although we as a species tend to outlive dogs, cats, mice, and chimpanzees, we can also differ a great deal from one another in the lengths of our lives. Now and then we see a newspaper article about a fifty-year-old marathon runner who, despite appearing to be as healthy as a horse, died of a heart attack after his race. On the other hand, it wasn't long ago that the comedian George Burns died at the age of one hundred after years of smoking cigars and living the high life in Hollywood. Doctors have never been able to fully explain these seemingly unfair anomalies.

Certainly it is common to attribute long life to "good genes," and heredity does play a part in determining life span. However, studies of identical twins have shown that genes are only about 25 percent of what determines exactly how long we live. In fact, research tells us that most of us have roughly the same chance of living to be eighty years old, regardless of how long our parents or grandparents lived. What is it then that changes in our bodies as we age such that our organs begin to fail and we eventually die? Does something necessary for life in our body run out, or does something toxic begin to build up? How forgiving is our body when we deprive it of the nutrients it needs or abuse it with unhealthy diets and substance abuse?

Beyond the assumption that the far limits of human life span are programmed into our genes, there are many theories as to why, in far too many cases, aging and death occur prematurely. By and large these are variations of the same theme. That is, that it results from the slow but steady accumulation of damage to proteins, fatty components of cell membranes, mitochondria, and DNA. The major culprit is oxidation, which is nothing less than the subtle but pervasive biological equivalent of rust. Other contributors are excesses of poorly chaperoned fat and sugar in the body. The collection of fat in places in the cell where it doesn't belong disturbs the orderly process of energy production in the mitochondria. When cells are flooded with glucose, proteins become disabled by chemical bonding with wayward sugar molecules. Lack of needed antioxidants and other nutrients in the diet and exposure to toxins that hamper cells in their fight to protect themselves add further to the processes of disintegration. Cells thus damaged can no longer defend themselves against the ravages of oxidation, which only accelerates the cycle of destruction. Some cells in the brain and other tissues bow out gracefully through the process of apoptosis. Others limp along in a state of disarray and suboptimal function. Damaged cells trip alarms, and the body marshals the only forces it knows by which to

---

apes, elephants, whales, and porpoises is only one of many possible evolutionary advantages of longevity. Population density, the likelihood of running into a mate, food supply, size, predators, and other factors may also determine such advantage.

defend itself. Inflammation, stress, and "fight or flight" mechanisms are triggered into action. Unfortunately, like firemen who tear through the roof to put out the fire in the attic, these mechanisms of defense themselves can become sources of damage and destruction. Thus, a growing consensus among scientists is that the length of our lives depends upon the complex interplay of genetic factors with diet, stress, activity, rest, exposure to environmental toxins and diseases, and other aspects of life that are matters of choice. For most of us, the same interplay between genes and lifestyle choices also determines whether or not we develop dementia.

CHANGES IN THE BRAIN AND MENTAL FUNCTION IN NORMAL AGING

It is likely that dementia has always been part of the human experience. Dementia in the elderly has been described in ancient Egyptian texts. The Greeks wrote extensively about the mind and the decline in its powers with age. The Greek philosopher Pythagoras believed that the mind began to deteriorate around the age of sixty-three. Hippocrates also considered dementia to be a normal and unavoidable effect of aging. However, even in ancient times, there was plenty of evidence that wisdom and intelligence did not necessarily dim with advancing years. The citizens of the Greek city-state Sparta were advised and led by a council of elders all over the age of sixty. Socrates, who was sentenced to die at the age of seventy by drinking hemlock due to his having "corrupted the young," continued to teach up until the day he died. Sophocles, a contemporary of Hippocrates, wrote his last great play, *Oedipus at Colonus*, at the age of ninety.

Losses in certain aspects of mental function do occur with advancing age. Nonetheless, many aging individuals maintain good mental function into their eighties or nineties. The consensus among physicians is that disabling decreases in function are *not* normal, and the dismissal of severe forgetfulness and confusion as simply an effect of aging is incorrect. It is prudent in such cases to consider the possibility of a dementing illness and to devise a treatment plan to reverse the condition or, at least, to slow its progression.

The most common and predictable effect of normal aging on mental performance is a decrease in the speed of cognitive processing. The elderly do not think as fast as the young. Their reaction times are slower, and they take longer to solve mental problems and to learn new things. The ability to pay attention is retained in aging. The normal elderly can focus on a task and work through it as well as younger people. It is being able to divide attention, in other words, to multitask, that becomes more difficult with age. However, to some extent this may be a matter of lacking the speed of cognitive processing necessary to manage multiple sources of information.

Older people also tend to lose what is called cognitive flexibility. In the laboratory, cognitive flexibility is measured as the ability to successfully continue a task after the instructions are changed in the middle of the test. In real life, a lack of cognitive flexibility might be reflected as difficulty in adapting to new ways of doing things, new tools, or new environments. Of course, one might argue that sticking to the "tried and true" has its benefits and that there may even be some biological advantage to being set in one's ways.

In normal aging there is increasing difficulty with new, nonverbal, visuo-spatial problems, such as copying complex designs or solving mazes. An example from everyday life would be that a normal elderly person is likely to have more difficulty than a young person going into an unfamiliar hardware store and locating items on a list of things to purchase. Another example is that elderly people aren't quite as facile as young people in planning routes of travel using road maps.

In normal aging, abstract thinking remains fairly intact. An example of abstract thinking is explaining the meaning of a common proverb, such as "People who live in glass houses shouldn't throw stones." A normal individual in our culture, regardless of age, should be able to explain that this is said when someone criticizes another person while being guilty of the same fault themselves. It has nothing to do with stones, glass, or architecture. However, those who have lost their capacity for abstract thinking are quite likely to explain that a person who lives in a glass house shouldn't throw stones because they'll break all the windows. Although they would be correct, this explanation is an example of concrete thinking and a sign of diminished cognitive function. The normal elderly are able to correctly explain this proverb. The normal elderly are also able to exercise the same type of conceptual thinking by explaining what they would do if they found an unmailed letter on the sidewalk or saw smoke coming out of the window of a neighbor's house. They should also have no difficulty describing the proper course of action to take in common situations of real life, such as what to do if a health problem evolves or if their car begins to show signs of needing repair.

Although the physiological mechanisms by which we lay down and retrieve memories have been the focus of intense study by neuroscientists for the past twenty-five years, much of the process of human memory remains a mystery. Nonetheless, what is clear is that the ability to remember what has recently occurred tends to diminish with age. Among the most poignant depictions of the vagaries of memory that come with aging was made by Mark Twain,[4] who near the end of his life remarked, "When I was younger I could remember anything, whether it happened or not; but my faculties are decaying now and soon I shall be so I cannot remember any but the things that never happened." Fortunately, for most people the reality is not so grim as that.

Most of us see memory as simply the ability to call to mind things that have happened in the past. However, cognitive neuroscientists who study the mind have defined many types and components of memory. In both normal aging and dementia, these various types of memory can be affected differently. Memory is generally categorized as declarative or procedural. Declarative memory involves the storage of information that can be talked about or described in some fashion. Procedural memory is the storage of information about how to do something, such as playing the piano or knitting a sweater. Usually, these are motor skills that are learned by repetition, not necessarily by thinking something through. As in the classic case of the golfer who loses his swing by trying to describe it, declarative and procedural memory can be separate or even at odds with each other. Procedural memory is quite enduring with age and can be retained even in individuals with obvious dementia. A common example is the elderly man who still successfully drives his car, but is unable to find his way to the drug store or ends up lost and confused in a town a hundred miles away from his home. Whereas procedural memory tends to be maintained with normal aging, certain types of declarative memory can suffer.

Declarative memory can be further categorized into semantic and episodic memory. Semantic memory is the ability to recall basic, commonly shared knowledge about the world. Examples would be knowing that in the United States we drive on the right side of the road or that soap and water are useful to clean dirty hands. Language itself falls in this category, as the meaning of words is stored in semantic memory. Episodic memory is the recall of specific events that individuals themselves have experienced. People's knowledge of who they voted for in the last election or what they had for breakfast this morning is retained in episodic memory.

Although it is useful to categorize memories into semantic and episodic, there is no compelling reason to see these two forms of memory as be-

---

4. Mark Twain was the pen name of the great American humorist Samuel Langhorne Clemens (November 30, 1835–April 21, 1910).

ing completely distinct in the mechanisms by which they are placed in or retrieved from the brain. To a large extent, it is how important a piece of information is and how often it is needed that tends to make it semantic versus episodic in character. Knowing the meaning of the phrase "dependent children" or the fact that you yield to the car on your right at a four-way stop sign are far more important than recalling whether you had oatmeal or ham and eggs for breakfast on any particular morning. On the other hand, certain memories that are personal, and thus categorized as episodic, may for all practical purposes be semantic in character. For example, I remember the telephone number of the house I grew up in in Kansas City as readily as I remember to ask for a spoon rather than a fork when I have been served a bowl of chicken soup.

Semantic memory remains largely intact in normal aging. For example, vocabulary usually remains strong. The normal elderly have no problem providing the meaning of words presented to them. They read and understand written material without difficulty. They may at times have some difficulty finding a correct word to say. When asked to name an object in a picture, they are more likely than young people to not recall the right name or to report the "tip of my tongue" phenomenon. However, if supplied with the correct word, they immediately recognize it as the word for which they were searching.

It is important that semantic memory remains largely intact, as it is part of the basis of the wisdom acquired with old age. From an evolutionary perspective, the wisdom that comes with age is probably the reason that human beings live so far beyond their reproductive years. Elderly people's knowledge and understanding of life and human behavior give their young a tremendous advantage in their own learning of how to survive and prosper in the world. Unfortunately, while an elderly person may be able to explain at length the benefits of giving the maitre d' of a restaurant a nice tip to ensure good service at dinner, he may be more likely to tip him twice, having forgotten that he had already done so. The latter error is due to the fact that episodic, more than semantic, memory can begin to suffer with age.

An important distinction to make in episodic memory is between recognition and recall. It is not uncommon for normal elderly people to drive perfectly well to the grocery store, but forget where they parked their cars. If they forget where they parked, this would be termed an inability to *recall*. If, after finding the car, they then remember parking at that spot, it would be said that they retained *recognition*. If they remain oblivious to having made the decision to park there in the first place, then they lack both recall and recognition, which is a sign of significant decline.

Another type of episodic memory that can be affected by age is working memory. Examples of working memory are the ability to remember a phone number long enough to make a call after retrieving the number from the directory or remembering instructions to perform a task of several steps. Working memory remains fairly intact with age. Deficits do appear if a list of numbers or objects to remember is too long or if there are distractions at the time the list is presented to memorize. In fact, one of the memory functions most vulnerable to aging is called secondary memory. This is the ability to remember newly learned information after attention has been directed toward other mental tasks. Some studies suggest that the function of secondary memory may decline as early as the fourth or fifth decade of life. Secondary memory is often studied in the laboratory by having subjects remember lists of words and then distracting them by having them fill in forms or solve simple puzzles before testing their recall of the list. In real life, it may reflect items to be purchased at the grocery store that would have more wisely been jotted down in a list rather than committed to memory. Driving to the store and finding a parking place would be distracters that might interfere with remembering what was on that list. A similar form of memory, called prospective memory, is the ability to remember an intention to do something later. It is the type of memory that gets jogged by the old method of tying a string around your finger. It is another form of episodic memory that tends to suffer with age.

It is important to point out that what is generally seen as a loss of function may in some cases merely be a change in the way the mind works. For example, a study recently found that normal elderly subjects and young college students respond differently when presented with reading selections that are interspersed with distractions, such as insertions of seemingly unrelated words and phrases. The young subjects were able to ignore those distractions and plow through the reading material more quickly. In comparison with the older subjects, they were also better able to recall details of the material that they had been led to believe were most important. The older subjects slowed down during the sections of distraction and did not perform as well on what they had been told was the primary task. However, much to the surprise of the researchers, the older subjects were better able to consider the significance of the "unimportant" distracting words and phrases when both groups were later quizzed about them. It is as if the young people simply ignored the distractions, whereas the older people, perhaps from experience, had been able to see that what may seem like simple distractions may often be important clues about what is really going on in the world. This ability to be cautious about what is really important and true may be yet another reflection of what we refer to as wisdom.

Although the elderly may have more difficulty learning new material and retaining it if distracted by other things, once they thoroughly commit this information to memory, the normal elderly can recall it nearly as well as young people. In the so-called *old* old, that is, people in their eighties and nineties, there tends to be accelerating losses in the ability to lay down and retrieve episodic memories. However, even in that age group, there can be considerable individual differences among people, and some can retain surprisingly good memory function.

An interesting and extremely common feature of dementia is an individual remembering events from childhood, but not being able to recall events from the previous day. This can seem puzzling and incongruous to family members, who tend to view those recollections from so long ago as evidence of the strength rather than the weakness of memory. However, this seemingly paradoxical phenomenon is simply an example of the fact that the primary problem in dementia, especially forms such as Alzheimer's in which the hippocampus is damaged by amyloid deposition, is the forming of new memories and not the retrieval of memories that are already held in storage in the brain. There does also come a time later in the progression of dementia when the retrieval of memory is also impaired, and sad and disturbing events such as forgetting a spouse's name or the names of children can begin to occur.

THE TIME COURSE OF CHANGE IN COGNITIVE FUNCTION

One of the most well-known and widely quoted studies of the effects of aging on cognitive function is the Seattle Longitudinal Study, which was led by Dr. K. Warner Schaie. In this study, more than five thousand people were followed for as long as thirty-five years and tested every seven years to reveal age-related changes in their abilities to use their minds. Among the areas of cognitive function studied were reasoning, spatial orientation, perceptual speed, numeric ability, verbal ability, and verbal memory.

One of the major findings of this study was that for the majority of people, there is little if any loss of cognitive function before the age of sixty. In fact, between the ages of twenty-five and sixty, many people show improvements in some of the ways they use their minds. The only function that doesn't improve during those years of life is the ability to work with numbers. The only striking loss is the inexorable decrease in the speed of perceptual processing, which can be seen as early as the age of thirty.

By the age of sixty-seven, most individuals reach a plateau in their cognitive functions, and may begin to enter the initial stages of decline. This becomes more evident by the early seventies and quite clear by the early eighties. However, as pointed out by Schaie, this decline in function can be quite gradual, and even at age eighty-one, fewer than half of the participants had shown significant decreases in function over the previous seven years. By the age of eighty-eight, deficits in numeric ability are often dramatic, and there are usually quite obvious decreases in episodic memory and the ability to solve problems involving spatial orientation and logic. Again, however, if the deficits in speed of processing are taken into account, even these seemingly dramatic changes in function may be seen as less severe.

Perhaps the most important finding of the Seattle study is that there can be substantial differences among people in the ways that aging affects the mind. Whereas some people show clear evidence of decline in their sixties, others maintain high levels of cognitive function even into their eighties and nineties. Although they are exceptions rather than the rule, there are many historical examples of extraordinary achievements in old age. Frank Lloyd Wright, rightfully considered the greatest American architect, lived to the age of ninety-one and continued to design buildings in the last years of his life. Luigi Cornaro, the Renaissance writer of advice for healthy living, wrote the last of his four treatises on health at the age of ninety-five. Anna Mary Robertson "Grandma" Moses continued to paint successfully at over one hundred years of age. The French chemist Michel-Eugène Chevreul, considered to be the father of the science of gerontology, did not take up his study of aging until he was in his nineties. He published his last scientific paper at the age of 102.

PHYSICAL CHANGES IN THE AGING BRAIN

Hippocrates was modern in his belief that the brain is the source of the mind. He believed it gave rise to joy, sorrow, wisdom, and knowledge, as well as delirium and madness. Yet, in Hippocrates' time, and for thousands of years after him, the workings of the brain and mind remained in the realm of gods, spirits, and other unseen forces. It wasn't until the Renaissance and Age of Enlightenment that anatomical studies of the brain began to reveal that the brain was an organ similar to other organs in the body. Although the brain is mysterious in its ability to generate intangible thoughts and feelings, like any other organ, it is subject to deterioration of its substance and structure. It came to be recognized that damage to brain tissue was responsible for changes in mental function, madness, melancholy, and dementia.

Age does bring structural and functional changes to the brain. Such changes are normal and expected. Some age-related changes in the brain are large and obvious enough to be seen by the modern techniques of computerized axial tomography (CAT scan) or magnetic resonance imaging (MRI). These computer-driven techniques generate detailed three-dimensional pictures of the brain that can be viewed in thinly sliced sections to reveal to the naked eye lesions as small as a few millimeters. Other changes are visible only under the microscope. Still others appear at the submicroscopic molecular level, and sophisticated techniques of biochemistry must be used to elucidate them. Depending on the type of change, and where in the brain these changes occur, the mind and behavior of an individual can be altered.

Structural Changes

Around the age of fifty, there begin to be decreases in the overall size and weight of the brains of normal individuals. Thereafter, the decrease in size of the brain progresses at a rate of about 2–3 percent per decade. These changes appear in images of the brain as flattening and shrinking of the gyri, which are the rope-like mounds of tissue that coil across the surface of the brain, and in increases in the widths of the sulci, which are the valleys that separate the gyri. There are also enlargements of the ventricles, which are the four fluid-filled spaces that lie within the brain. The age-related loss of volume of brain tissue includes both gray and white matter. Gray matter consists of the bodies of nerve cells. White matter is formed from the axons of those nerve cells, which serve as communication lines from one part of the brain to another. White matter is white due to the fatty insulating material that wraps around the axons to insure clear, crisp signals from cell to cell.

Although it is reasonable to suspect that shrinkage in the size of the brain would result in decreases in cognitive function, there is no clear relationship between mere size of the brain and mental capability. In fact, studies have shown that 15 percent of adults over the age of sixty with normal cognitive function may also have moderate to severe shrinkage of brain size. The classical explanation for the shrinkage of gray matter volume in aging brains has been loss of neurons. However, recent scientific studies have shown that actual loss of neurons may not be as severe as was once thought. To some extent, loss of volume may be due to the mere shrinking in size of some nerve cells, and not necessarily their death and disappearance. Furthermore, there is no evidence that this shrinkage in size dramatically alters the activity of those neurons.

Age-related changes do not occur homogenously throughout the brain. Certain areas are more strongly affected than others. It has been suggested that areas that are relatively new in the evolution of the brain are the ones most vulnerable to the adverse effects of aging. The newer areas of the brain tend to be the ones most responsible for the uniquely human qualities of the mind, such as judgment, creativity, and abstract thinking. The prefrontal cortex, which is uniquely well developed in humans, is one of the areas most vulnerable to age-related loss of volume.

The prefrontal cortex is an extraordinarily complex system of neurons, and destruction of this part of the brain through injury or stroke can result in dramatic changes in behavior and function. However, in normal aging the moderate degree of tissue loss in the prefrontal cortex causes only subtle changes in cognitive function. For example, whereas severe damage to this area substantially reduces the ability to name objects in pictures, normal elderly people generally perform this task without much difficulty. It is only when the difficulty of such a task is heightened, for example, by showing test objects from an unusual perspective, such as a bird's eye view rather than eye level, that deficits in performance become apparent. Similarly, while the prefrontal cortex plays an important role in processing episodic and working memory, deficits in these memory functions become apparent in normal elderly subjects only when the information to remember becomes unusually long or if distractions are added to complicate the task. It is quite likely that the gradual, age-related losses in the prefrontal cortex can be compensated for by changes in the activity of areas that are less affected by age.

The hippocampus, an evolutionarily older part of the brain, is less affected by age, per se. However, it is exquisitely sensitive to factors such as stress, inadequate blood supply, hypoxia, low blood sugar, and psychiatric illnesses such as major depression. Such factors may be at least partially responsible for inconsistencies in the literature concerning the degree to which the hippocampus is subject to loss of tissue in aging. The hippocampus does shrink with age, but there is evidence that in normal individuals this may not be prominent until they reach their seventies. It must also be noted that while the hippocampal function is critical for the laying down of new memories, there is no clear relationship between hippocampal volume and the ability to perform tasks of memory.

Up until recently, it was thought that neurons in the brain were not replaced when they die, and therefore that the death of neurons invariably led to a net loss in the number of these cells. However, it has been found that new neurons are produced in the brain. This process is called neurogenesis. The hippocampus is one of the major areas in which neurogenesis takes place. One reason for shrinkage of the hippocampus in states of stress is disruption of neurogenesis by high levels of the stress hormone cortisol. Cortisol levels are increased in major depression and Alzheimer's dementia. Cortisol may also be increased in metabolic syndrome, an increasingly common condition that I will later focus on in some detail.

The cingulate and entorhinal cortices are other areas that are slightly reduced in size with aging. However, in Alzheimer's dementia, there is substantial cell loss in those two areas as well as in the hippocampus. The cingulate cortex plays an important role in attention and the focusing of motivation, which become disturbed in moderate and severe dementia. The entorhinal cortex plays a critical role in the sense of smell. This is likely to explain why the loss of ability to recognize and name odors is an early sign of Alzheimer's dementia. The degree of loss of volume in those areas may serve as a means to differentiate the normal losses of aging from the ravages of neurodegenerative diseases.

Microscopic Changes

Whereas CAT scans show shrinkage of certain areas of the brain to be a normal part of aging, microscopic evaluation reveals additional age-related changes in brain tissue. These changes appear in older people who may be entirely free of any evidence of dementia, and they have been thought to represent the normal aging process. Microscopic brain lesions called neurofibrillary tangles and neuritic plaques are the primary diagnostic markers of Alzheimer's dementia. Both neurofibrillary tangles, consisting of *tau* protein, and neuritic plaques, consisting of the abnormal protein *beta amyloid*, can be found in the aging brains of normal individuals. The primary difference between normal brains and those of patients with Alzheimer's dementia is the number of those lesions and the areas in which they proliferate.

It has been reported that roughly 30 percent of people over the age of seventy-five who are free of symptoms of dementia have moderate numbers of neuritic amyloid plaques in the cerebral cortex of their brains. However, they have about half of the number of such plaques as are usually seen in the brains of age-matched patients with Alzheimer's dementia. In some areas of the brain, there is little difference between demented and non-demented subjects in the number of plaques. The differences are most noticeable in the hippocampus and prefrontal cortex, which play important roles in memory and executive functions. In Alzheimer's dementia, these areas become choked with amyloid plaques.

Neurofibrillary tangles are more common than plaques in the brains of elderly people, including those without dementia. They are often found in and around the hippocampus. However, among non-demented subjects with tangles were individuals as old as eighty-eight who had brains virtually free of neuritic amyloid plaques. Thus, tangles alone may not to be sufficient to cause loss of cognitive function, and the plaques and tangles that have been seen as markers of Alzheimer's dementia may not necessarily be caused by the same underlying problems. On the other hand, recent studies are showing that neurofibrillary tangles may play a more important role in the erosion of cognitive function than was previously suspected. Several new medications that specifically decrease the amount of existing tangles of tau protein and prevent further development of these neurofibrillary tangles in the brains of patients with Alzheimer's dementia can improve cognitive function and prevent further decline.

Because age is the factor most clearly related to Alzheimer's dementia, it has at times been wondered whether the plaques, tangles, and lesions of Alzheimer's and other neurodegenerative dementias reflect disease processes or are simply early presentations of normal patterns of aging. Similarly, it has been suspected that anyone who lived long enough would eventually develop dementia and lesions in their brains similar to those seen in the neurodegenerative disorders. At times, the distinctions between degenerative illness and normal aging can be difficult to make. Nonetheless, the preponderance of data shows that dementia is an abnormal condition and that normal aging does not entail amyloid plaques, neurofibrillary tangles, degeneration of brain tissue, or serious loss of cognitive functions.

There has recently been a report in the well-regarded scientific journal *Neurobiology of Aging* of a woman who lived to be 115 years old. When tested at the age of 112, she scored extremely well on the Mini-Mental State Examination, which is a standard screening tool for diagnosing dementia. Her score of 27 out of 30 was well above the scores that would lead to suspicion of dementia. She was retested two years later and scored 26. Even in the last months of her life she maintained an extraordinary degree of cognitive function, and at autopsy she was found to be virtually free of the changes in the brain generally associated with Alzheimer's and other neurodegenerative dementias. This woman, and other centenarians who have been studied and found to have relatively intact mental faculties and brains, gives clear evidence for the fact that age, per se, does not unavoidably lead to degeneration of the brain and loss of cognitive function.

While even advanced age does not necessarily entail the development of plaques and tangles in brain tissue, there are individuals who do develop such lesions at young ages due to genetic abnormalities in brain chemistry. As if people with Down syndrome didn't suffer enough from mental retardation, they are also a group prone to developing plaques and tangles in their brains at very early ages. Patients with Down syndrome who live into their forties generally develop extensive deposition of amyloid in their brains and experience further decreases in their cognitive function consistent with a progressive dementia. Individuals with the severe familial form of Alzheimer's dementia tend to exhibit deposition of plaques and diminished cognitive function by the relatively early age of fifty, whereas those with the more common sporadic form of Alzheimer's do not display such signs until they are over sixty-five. All in all, it can be said that while age is a risk factor for the development of the neuritic plaques and neurofibrillary tangles that characterize Alzheimer's dementia, it is neither necessary nor sufficient for this to occur. Clearly, other factors are involved.

Changes in the health and function of blood vessels in the brain also tend to occur with aging. Some appear to be due to normal and expected aging processes and occur in both humans and animals. Capillaries are the smallest blood vessels in the brain. They are often wide enough to allow only a single red blood cell to slide through them. In most tissues, cells are either immediately adjacent or only one or two cell layers away from these vessels. In the normal elderly brain, the ratio between the number of neurons and the number of capillaries in brain tissue increases, which results in less oxygen and glucose getting to neurons, which require these vital nutrients. The endothelium, which is the specialized cellular lining of large and small arteries, becomes less responsive to demands for increased blood flow in active aging brains. This further impairs flow of nutrients.

Although adverse changes in blood vessels tend to occur even in the brains of normal elderly individuals, they are particularly marked among those with cardiovascular disease. This is often due to years of stress placed on these vessels by high blood pressure, inflammation, high cholesterol, high blood sugar, and oxidative stress. Amyloid, the same protein that deposits itself in plaques around neurons, may also accumulate in the walls of capillaries and small arteries. Those walls then become thick, stiff, more resistant to blood flow, and less able to meet the brain's changing demands for blood as it increases its activity. Hardening, narrowing, or outright blockage of arteries in the brain cause what is generally referred to as vascular dementia. Although tangles and plaques are thought to be the primary lesions of Alzheimer's dementia, many scientists are beginning to suspect that poor transfer of oxygen and glucose into the brain may also contribute to the development and progression of Alzheimer's and other neurodegenerative forms of dementia.

Amyloid plaques and neurofibrillary tangles are the primary features that characterize the brain tissue of sufferers of Alzheimer's dementia. However, pathologists who study the brain have described and named a wide variety of spots, discolorations, and darkened knots of proteins that can begin to appear in microscopic examination of the brain either as disease processes or simply as a part of normal aging.

All living cells produce waste products. In most cases, these wastes are excreted from the cell into the bloodstream and then either broken down or expelled from the body by the liver, lungs, or kidneys. However, as cells age, one waste product, called lipofuscin, begins to collect inside them. Lipofuscin consists primarily of degraded, oxidized fat molecules and partially oxidized proteins that cross-link and form knots of dark material that can neither be digested nor expelled by the cell. Instead, the cells store it away in vacuoles, which are basically the cells' trash cans. This is not just a human problem, nor is it due to unhealthy lifestyles. It is a largely unavoidable product of metabolism. Lipofuscin forms and accumulates in all living cells, whether in otter, osprey, or ophthalmologist, and the general rule is that the older the cell is, the more lipofuscin it will contain.

It is controversial whether the accumulation of lipofuscin poses a danger to living cells or if the ability to isolate and contain the substance is a clever and effective way for the cells to prevent damage from this cellular garbage. It is known that neurons in certain areas of the brain best able to resist loss of function from age-related degenerative processes also tend to be avid accumulators of lipofuscin. On the other hand, excessive accumulation of lipofuscin is generally seen in the retinas of patients with macular degeneration, an eye condition in which cell death in the retina leads to blindness. Thus, it is possible that brain cells would live longer and perform better without the extra burden of lipofuscin. Although lipofuscin cannot be entirely prevented from forming, it is known that antioxidants can slow the rate of its accumulation in cells. Its formation and accumulation may also be decreased by substances such as carnosine, a nutrient and natural substance in the body, which may prevent cross-linking of protein fragments and aid in the expulsion rather than accumulation of these wastes. Carnosine and a variety of substances with potent antioxidant effects are discussed in the chapter on herbs, vitamins, and nutraceuticals.

Hirano bodies are small, rod-shaped objects that can sometimes be seen in neurons of normal aging brains. They are often quite numerous in the brains of patients with Alzheimer's dementia. They contain fragments of various proteins that form the internal skeletal and transport systems of neurons. One protein, tau, is found in both Hirano bodies and the neurofibrillary tangles found in the brain tissue of patients with Alzheimer's disease. Because they can occur in normal individuals, it isn't clear if or how Hirano bodies might be related to dementia. Nonetheless, the abundance of Hirano bodies in the hippocampi of patients with Alzheimer's suggests they can contribute to memory deficits, as this area of the brain is critical for the laying down of memories.

It has been found that substances called advanced glycation endproducts, or AGEs, increase the rate of Hirano body formation. As I will later discuss, AGEs themselves are generated as a result of poorly controlled sugar metabolism and oxidative stress. Thus, it is likely that Hirano bodies are caused by the same aberrant conditions that are rampant in Alzheimer's and other degenerative brain disorders. Healthy diets that control blood sugar, maintain insulin sensitivity, and contain adequate levels of antioxidants may help prevent or at least minimize proliferation of Hirano bodies.

Lewy bodies are small spots that stain darkly when treated with agents that react with the brain protein called alpha-synuclein. These abnormal collections of synuclein are always present in patients who have Parkinson's disease and, by definition, those who have Lewy body dementia. However, they are also quite common in the brains of patients with Alzheimer's dementia. In one study it was reported that about 30 percent of Alzheimer's patients have Lewy bodies along with amyloid plaques and neurofibrillary tangles of tau protein in their brains at autopsy. However, Lewy bodies of tangled synuclein protein do not often appear during normal aging of the brain. Even in quite elderly populations, they are seen in less than 10 percent of individuals without diagnosed neurodegenerative disease.

Aside from spots and tangles that can appear in and around neurons, other age-related changes in brain tissue that can be seen under the microscope include structural changes in dendrites of neurons. "Dendrite" is derived from the Greek word for tree. Dendrites are branched tree-like structures that extend from the cell body of neurons to make connections with other neurons. The points of contact between neurons are called synapses, and they are sites at which chemical messages are transmitted from one neuron to another. The extent and complexity of the dendritic branching in brain tissue reflects the amount of information that gets shared among the residing neurons. The more branches and synapses a neuron possesses, the more information it can send, receive, and process.

The extent of dendritic branching tends to decrease with age, even among individuals without evidence of dementia. Some studies have shown that by the age of sixty there can be a 20 percent decrease in dendritic branching of cortical neurons. There are indications, however, that in spite of overall decreases in dendritic branching, neurons in the normal aged brain can still make up for losses or damage of neurons within certain areas of the brain by increasing the dendritic branching of intact adjacent neurons. Neurons of patients with Alzheimer's dementia are not able to generate such compensatory increases in dendritic branching. The growth and maintenance of the dendritic trees require the activity of various stimulating substances known collectively as neurotrophic factors. A number of pathological processes in the brain can interfere with the normal production of these factors. On the other hand, there are a variety of herbs and so-called nutraceuticals, which are often substances naturally produced in the body, that can stimulate their production. Although age results in decreases in the extent and complexity of dendritic branching, other processes, most notably high levels of cortisol in persistent states of stress, can cause similar adverse changes in neuronal structure. To some extent this may be due to inhibition of the synthesis of neurotrophic factors. There are indications that age and stress can interact to cause even more severe damage to dendrites.

Chemical Changes

Aging can also produce changes in chemistry and metabolism that are far too small to be seen under a microscope. Studies have shown that the aged brain does not use as much oxygen or glucose as the younger brain, and this corresponds to decreases in function in the affected areas of the brain. Some of the decreases in the metabolism of oxygen and glucose may be due to age-related decreases in the function of mitochondria in the brain. Mitochondria are the energy-producing units inside cells. They convert fuel, in the form of fat and glucose, into energy. The process of converting fuel to energy unleashes a number of dangerous by-products, including free radicals, which can severely damage the walls of mitochondria and other cellular structures. The cell depends on natural antioxidants and protective enzymes to protect itself from these highly reactive substances. Nonetheless, with time, it is inevitable that some damage will be done. It has long been known that mitochondrial function declines with age, and this is likely due to cumulative damage from free radicals. Although these adverse changes are normal, and occur in both human and animal brains, there are reasons to believe that the damage can be minimized with healthy diet and adequate supply of antioxidants.

The concentrations of many of the chemical messengers released from one neuron to another also decrease with age. These chemicals are called neurotransmitters, and among the ones that decrease with age are serotonin, dopamine, norepinephrine, and acetylcholine. Decreases in the various transmitters can contribute to adverse changes in both cognitive function and mood. Decreases in levels of serotonin and norepinephrine are associated with major depression. Decreases in the production of dopamine add to depressed mood and are known to be responsible for the movement disturbances of Parkinson's disease. Acetylcholine is profoundly reduced in Alzheimer's dementia, and most of the medications currently used to treat this illness act by increasing the availability of this neurotransmitter.

3

THE PRESENTATION AND DIAGNOSIS OF DEMENTIA

The most widely accepted definition of dementia, which can be found in the American Psychiatric Association's *Diagnostic and Statistical Manual of Mental Disorders, Fourth Edition* (DSM-IV), is a condition of loss of memory, accompanied by impairment of decision making or personality change. To be considered as dementia, such changes in mental function must be severe enough to interfere significantly with an individual's work, social activities, or relationships with others. Although Alzheimer's disease is often thought of as being synonymous with dementia, there are, in fact, many different types and causes of dementia. They are all neurological disorders that arise from degeneration of brain tissue. They differ from one another in the underlying nature of the degeneration and in the area of the brain where losses of tissue tend to occur. These differences, in turn, cause them to present in somewhat different fashion from one another and to progress in different manners. Distinguishing one form of dementia from another is important because these different illnesses can require different types of treatment to relieve symptoms or to at least slow the disease process. This is where the trained eye of the neurologist, geriatrician, or psychiatrist is critical for proper diagnosis and treatment.

Alzheimer's disease is the cause of just over half of all cases of dementia. Other types of dementia include vascular, Lewy body, and frontotemporal in roughly that order of frequency. Rarer forms of dementia, which I will not discuss in detail, include progressive supranuclear palsy,

Huntington's chorea, and Creutzfeldt-Jakob disease. There are also a number of conditions that mimic dementia, but unlike the neurodegenerative forms of dementia, they can be reversed if diagnosed and treated in early stages. These conditions include major depression, normal pressure hydrocephalus, sleep apnea, thyroid hormone deficiency, and deficiencies of vitamin B_{12}, folic acid, and other essential nutrients. If not caught early, these potentially reversible conditions can cause irreversible damage and dementia.

The diagnosis of dementia is essentially a three-step process. First, there must be suspicion from the presentation of the patient, their complaints, or complaints of the family that the individual is suffering changes in cognitive function consistent with dementia. The second step is to rule out other medical and psychiatric conditions that may mimic dementia. Finally, if signs and symptoms of dementia are present and cannot be explained by another condition, then it is necessary to determine what type of dementia is present and what the best method of treatment should be.

PRESENTATION

The presentation of an illness is simply the way patients appear when they first come to be evaluated for possible illness. This includes not only how patients look and feel, but also the manner and circumstances of their arrival at the doctor's office. In my own practice, some patients will arrange on their own to come and be evaluated for what they fear may be dementia. Others ask on the spur of the moment, during a regularly scheduled appointment, if I think they might be developing Alzheimer's disease. Now and then one will ask me if they have "old-timer's disease," which I always find a sadly endearing question.

There has been a great deal written about the meaning and significance of patients' beliefs that they are losing their memory. This kind of complaint is so common that it has even been given a name in the medical literature, subjective cognitive impairment, or SCI. Not everyone with SCI has dementia. People with severe or even moderate dementia are often oblivious to their loss of cognitive function. Consequently, SCI is relatively uncommon among this group of patients. However, it stands to reason that at some point between being normal and starting to experience significant loss of memory, people can be exquisitely aware of their problem. SCI is sometimes seen in people with mild dementia and more commonly in a condition that is referred to as mild cognitive impairment.

When people experience memory deficits that do not significantly interfere with their social or work life, and thus do not fulfill the criteria to be called dementia, they are said to have mild cognitive impairment, or MCI.[1] In many cases, MCI progresses to dementia, but in other cases it does not. Many experts believe that subjective recognition of memory loss is fairly common in people with MCI. However, it is also known that some with MCI, whether out of pride, denial, or lack of awareness, will not complain about it. Thus clinicians and family members should keep a low threshold for suspicions about loss of memory.

With the exception of rare cases of genetically linked early-onset dementia, the vast majority of cases of dementia are diagnosed in people who are in their sixties or older. Thus, unless there is a family history of early-onset dementia, the most likely cause of forgetfulness and difficulty concentrating in a person under the age of sixty is major depression, an anxiety disorder, or some other psychiatric illness. There is, in fact, evidence in the medical literature that patients under sixty-five who volunteer concerns about memory loss and suspect they might have dementia are more likely to be suffering depression and anxiety than true dementia. In some cases, severe depression can produce forgetfulness, slowness of thought, and changes in mood that are very similar to dementia. This phenomenon is sometimes referred to as pseudodementia. When memory loss is due to depression, the loss reverses with successful treatment of the depressive disorder.

Although major depression can cause genuine difficulties with memory, it is often the case that patients with depression merely *think* that they have lost their memory. Many such people are found to have normal memory function when tested by standard methods. This self-perception of being unable to remember is probably a reflection of the negative, self-deprecating way of seeing the world that tends to arise in states of depression. Of course, a person can have both depression and MCI or dementia. In fact, it is quite common for people in the early stages of dementia to experience depression. Thus, a diagnosis of major depression in no way rules out the possibility of also having dementia.

A common presentation of a patient with true dementia is a somewhat confused, mildly annoyed individual brought to the doctor's office by concerned family members. Almost invariably, it is the family's idea to bring the patient in, and the patient would much prefer to be elsewhere. It is

---

1. Some authorities discuss forms of MCI that involve diminution of cognitive functions other than memory, such as deficiencies in decision making or subtle losses of self-restraint in social situations. These conditions are referred to as non-amnestic MCI.

not unusual for people in mild or moderate stages of dementia to lack the ability to be objective about changes in their cognitive performance. They may underestimate their problems and deny or be completely oblivious to any loss of cognitive function. For that reason, it is often the reports of family and friends that provide the clearest evidence of dementia in a patient. It is an interesting observation among doctors that many patients with mild or moderate dementia will display the so-called head-turning sign in response to questions during the office evaluation of their cognitive function. When asked simple questions such as the date, their street address, medications they take, or how many grandchildren they have, they tend not to answer, but rather to turn their heads toward their spouses or other family members hoping to get the correct answer from them. I have quite often witnessed this phenomenon.

Unfortunately, it is often serious incidents, such as repeatedly leaving the stove on and burning pots of food, getting lost at the mall, or being swindled by a predatory telemarketer that lead a family to bring the patient in for evaluation. Such extreme behaviors tend to suggest that a dementing process is already well under way. It is the milder, more subtle disturbances of so-called activities of daily living, often referred to as ADLs, that can help a family, a patient, and a doctor come to suspect dementia early in the disease process. When family members express even vague suspicion about their loved one's cognitive function, it is important to obtain their help in taking an inventory of the performance of ADLs, such as personal hygiene, housekeeping, shopping, cooking, managing medications, and other basic skills of independent life. The family should also be asked about changes in personality and behavior, such as suspiciousness, inappropriate sexual comments, rudeness, or any other uncharacteristic behaviors that could indicate subtle changes in brain function. Such an inventory is also advisable when an elderly person is seen for a regularly scheduled checkup. Any indications of deficits should prompt the physician to perform a more focused screening for dementia. A poor performance in the dementia screening test should trigger more detailed studies to confirm the existence, and identify the type and stage, of a dementing illness.

OFFICE SCREENING TESTS FOR DEMENTIA

One of the best screening tools that doctors use to get a sense of a patient's level of cognitive function is the Mini-Mental State Examination, or MMSE. This extremely useful and widely used test was developed in 1975 by Dr.

Marshal Folstein, and it is sometimes referred to as "the Folstein test." It can be performed in any doctor's office in only ten to fifteen minutes. The MMSE consists of eleven questions that evaluate the basic components of cognitive function, including orientation to time and place, working memory, short-term memory, attention, calculation, reading, writing, following commands, and ability to interpret and copy simple geometric forms.

Although not completely comprehensive or detailed in its conclusions, the MMSE has been proven to be accurate in revealing potential problems. There are 30 possible points to score in the test, and a score of 23 or less is suggestive of cognitive deficits. A score of 20 to 23 is consistent with mild dementia, 12 to 19 is consistent with moderate dementia, and any score below 12 suggests a severe dementia. The age and education of the patient must be taken into account when interpreting the MMSE score, as old age and little education can be expected to lower the score by a few points. For example, one task in the MMSE is to spell a word backward. Individuals who are poorly educated and not very good at spelling may be placed at an unfair disadvantage on this task. The astute clinician can take such factors into consideration when drawing conclusions from the MMSE.

Another easily performed screening test that is gaining popularity among clinicians is the Montreal Cognitive Assessment, or MOCA. Like the MMSE, it evaluates components of cognitive function, including visuospatial, executive, attention, naming, language, memory, and abstraction. There is impressive data showing that the MOCA may be more sensitive in revealing early indications of cognitive loss, including better recognition of mild cognitive impairment, than the MMSE. The MOCA is also thought to be less affected by age and education. Most physicians have been exposed to the MMSE in their training and are therefore probably more comfortable in using it. However, if you remain concerned about subtle changes in a loved one's cognitive function, you might mention to the doctor the possibility of using the MOCA rather than the MMSE to more finely discern what is going on.

A scale often used by doctors to help measure the severity and track the progression of dementia goes by the rather angelic name of the Blessed Dementia Scale. Although devised in 1968, by the British neuropsychologist Dr. Garry Blessed, it remains a useful tool in modern psychiatry and neurology. The primary value of the Blessed Scale versus the MMSE or the MOCA is that a large part of the score depends upon how well individuals are able to function in their daily lives and how they behave on a day-to-day basis. Input from family and caregivers is required to obtain the information. Points are added when ordinary activities such as being able to do household chores, deal with money, or feed oneself are deficient. Points are

also added if aberrant behaviors, such as sexual inappropriateness, uncharacteristic selfishness, or emotional hypersensitivity have been exhibited.
The higher the score, the more severe the dementia. The main drawback of
the Blessed Dementia Scale is that the skills evaluated and questions asked
are so basic and simple that the test has no ability to give indications that a
person might be suffering mild cognitive impairment or be in the earliest
stages of dementia.

A more recently developed testing scale with a grimmer title, the Global
Deterioration Scale, is similar to the Blessed Dementia Scale in gauging the
severity of dementia from information about individuals' level of functioning and behavior in their usual environment. The scale defines seven stages
ranging from stage 1, in which there are no deficits whatsoever, to stage 7,
in which there is little if any verbal ability, no control of bowel and bladder,
and a loss of basic motor skills, including the ability to walk and feed oneself. Overall, stage 7 of the Global Deterioration Scale is described as the
state in which "the brain appears to no longer be able to tell the body what
to do." The presence and severity of dementia is determined by comparing
the patient's behaviors with those described in the scale and determining
which stage the patient's level of function most closely matches. Like the
Blessed Scale, it is not terribly useful for discovering subtle deficits or warning about the possibility of mild cognitive impairment.

The usual practice for gauging the degree of dementia in a patient is to
categorize his or her symptoms into stages of mild, moderate, or severe
dementia. This distinction is important to help provide patients and their
families some sense of what to expect in terms of prognosis and the time
course of the illness and to determine the level of supervision a patient
might need to remain safe. It is also critical for planning medical treatment,
as some medications are approved by the Federal Drug Administration for
only certain stages of illness.

A low score on a cognitive function test simply informs the doctor that
the patient is not thinking well. This could be due to dementia; however, it
might also be due to depression, an infection, or a metabolic disturbance.
Something as simple as poor eyesight or loss of hearing can also adversely
affect the test scores. I recall evaluating a 101-year-old man on the medical
floor of the hospital where I worked. He had complained of abdominal pain
in the middle of the night and had been rushed off from his nursing home to
our hospital a hundred miles away. An MMSE performed by the admitting
physician on the evening of his arrival had suggested that he was severely
demented. In fact, the unfortunate man was blind and nearly deaf. He had
no way of knowing where he was or what day or month it was because no one

had bothered to tell him. He couldn't hear the instructions of the test and couldn't see to perform the tests of reading and copying figures. After speaking with him for a few minutes, it became clear to me that he was far more cognitively intact than anyone had suspected from the perfunctory MMSE.

Although the final score of the MMSE or MOCA is determined entirely by how many questions are answered correctly, I have found that the manner in which an answer is given can be more telling than whether or not it is the right answer. For example, manner can sometimes be helpful in discerning whether a patient suffers dementia or if they are primarily depressed. If I ask patients with depression to perform a task such as spelling a word backward, they are likely to answer, in a slow monotone fashion, "No, I can't do that." However, if I cajole them into trying, they are often able to do it perfectly well. On the other hand, a person with dementia but without depression may quickly and even cheerfully say "Yes," if I ask them if they would be able to perform that task. However, when I ask them to go ahead and do it, they are often totally lost. Similarly, if I ask depressed patients if they know what year this is, they may say, "I don't know." When I ask if they would just guess, their guesses are often correct. Patients with dementia may quickly say "Yes," but when I ask them to go ahead and tell me what year it is, they can not.

A perfect score on the MMSE or MOCA does not guarantee that a patient is free of dementing illness. A well-educated, sixty-year-old bank executive may be showing signs of cognitive dysfunction by changes in personality and not performing at her usual high level in complicated financial transactions. However, she may still perform quite well on the relatively easy and straightforward MMSE or MOCA tests. It is also important to consider what types of questions are missed in the tests. Although a score of 27 may be considered normal, if a sixty-year-old man misses all three points in the test of short-term memory, I would be concerned, particularly if recent changes in behavior and performance of ADLs had led the patient or his family to arrange an appointment for evaluation.

If a test of cognitive function score is low, or if a "normal" score does not allay persistent concerns about dementia, it is important to perform other tests to determine what is causing the changes in cognitive function. It may be worthwhile to undergo a more complete battery of tests performed by a specialist in the field, that is, a neuropsychologist. These professionals are able to discern subtle or isolated changes in cognitive function that might not appear in the usual office screening tests. Confusing cases may also be illuminated by brain imaging studies and laboratory studies of blood, urine, or cerebrospinal fluid, as I will soon discuss.

ALTERNATIVE TESTS

A very interesting and potentially useful diagnostic test for dementia has been developed out of findings that patients with Alzheimer's and Lewy body dementias have difficulty identifying odors. This difficulty is partly due to losses of cognitive function that make it difficult to come up with the name connected with the odor. However, there is also evidence that areas of brain that process the sense of smell suffer neurodegenerative damage very early on in the development of these illnesses. There is even some evidence that deficits in the identification of odors can be seen in people with MCI, although these deficits are considered to be very modest and not reliable for diagnosis.

A method of testing identification of odors is to present the patient with ten to sixteen different odors, such as orange, cinnamon, banana, licorice, turpentine, garlic, coffee, and other easily recognizable odors, on blank cards. The number of odors that cannot be identified usually parallels the degree of severity of the dementia.[2] Two fairly obvious caveats that must be mentioned are to not test when the patient has a head cold or allergic rhinitis and to be certain that the odors to identify are culturally relevant to the individual being tested. For example, an individual from Southeast Asia might be able to identify the pungent smell of durian fruit, but not peppermint, due to differences in likelihood of having previously been exposed to the odor.

An interesting, although largely abandoned, method has been to measure the sensitivity of the pupil of the eye to administration of eye drops containing drugs that block activity at the acetylcholine receptor. Acetylcholine antagonists cause dilation of the pupils. This effect has been exploited by "bar girls" who would put drops of extract of the plant belladonna in their eyes. The drops dilate their pupils and make them seem more interested and interesting to male customers. Belladonna, in fact, translates into English as "beautiful woman." There have been indications that baseline deficits in acetylcholine activity in patients with Alzheimer's dementia are amplified when drugs that block acetylcholine receptors are taken. This same effect is seen when people with dementia take anticholinergic medications, such as diphenhydramine in over-the-counter sleeping pills, and react with severe confusion and delirium. The pupils in the eye are seen as literally a "window" to observe a person's sensitivity to anticholinergic substances.

---

2. There is interesting data showing that people who suffer schizophrenia also have difficulty identifying odors in this test. It is not exactly clear why this might be the case, but it is an active area of research.

However, while there is evidence that patients with Alzheimer's dementia do have a marked pupillary sensitivity to anticholinergic drugs, the response isn't specific enough to dementia to be diagnostic.

A group of physical signs that neurologists often look for in evaluating possible neurodegenerative disease are "frontal release" signs. These signs are essentially primitive, infantile reflexes that tend to re-emerge when higher, cortical inhibition of these once automatic responses begins to deteriorate. These are some of the most interesting and enigmatic diagnostic signs in medicine. The palmo-mental sign is a twitching of the chin that occurs in response to quickly and firmly dragging the thumbnail across the palm of one of the patient's outstretched hands. The glabellar sign is the patient's inability to keep from blinking when the examiner taps repeatedly on the forehead between the eyes. The grasp reflex is an involuntary closure of the patient's fingers around the fingers of the examiner as they are raked downward across the outstretched palms of the patient. In cases of significant frontal lobe damage, it is sometimes possible to elicit the rooting reflex, in which patients turn their heads to take the examiner's finger into their mouths when it has been stroked against their cheeks. This is reminiscent of the reflexes that guide infants' heads as they turn to take the nipple into their mouths to nurse.

Although fascinating, the diagnostic value of the frontal release signs has rightfully been called into question. Some perfectly normal people can exhibit some of these signs, particularly the palmo-mental sign. Moreover, an inability to elicit such signs cannot be used to rule out dementia or frontal lobe damage in individuals showing obvious signs of cognitive loss. Nonetheless, they can be important clues suggestive of neurodegeneration.

I vividly recall a "real life" frontal release sign that my father displayed after he began his descent into what I suspect was a form of frontotemporal dementia. I was visiting my parents back in Kansas City, and I was treating them to a new recipe I had for spaghetti sauce. As the pot of tomato paste, red wine, Italian sausage, garlic, and spices simmered on the stove, my father dipped in a spoon and brought it to his mouth to sample the taste. Perhaps due to the fact that my father had erroneously been under the impression that I was preparing beef stew rather than a slightly more tart spaghetti sauce, the moment the spoon entered his mouth he quite involuntarily twisted his face, wrinkled his nose, and puckered his lips as if he had just spooned the juice of a thousand lemons into his mouth. His face was the perfect picture of an infant who had just tasted something awful. Most remarkable was that from out of his contorted lips came the words, "That's really good!"

RULE OUT OTHER CAUSES

Medical science is advancing so rapidly that we are fast approaching the time when a simple blood test may reveal the presence of Alzheimer's disease or other forms of dementia. However, at present, the diagnosis of dementia is still made clinically, that is, by taking a good history of the patient's symptoms, exploring the family's history of dementia, and thoroughly evaluating the patient to determine what his or her level of cognitive function actually is. It should also be noted that the diagnosis of dementia is largely a diagnosis of exclusion. The doctor rules out factors such as major depression, head injury, hormone deficiencies, sleep apnea, infections, medication side effects, and other medical problems as being the cause of the altered mental status. If those possibilities are ruled out, then dementia remains as the likely cause of the deficits in cognitive function.

An essential part of the evaluation to rule out of possible medical causes of deterioration of cognitive function is a thorough physical examination. An experienced and observant clinician can appreciate signs indicative of medical problems that can be causing or contributing to cognitive dysfunction. Heart failure, liver disease, hormonal imbalances, and other illnesses all tend to present with specific physical signs that can provide clues as to possible physical problems underlying changes in cognitive function. An important part of such an examination is a thorough and systematic evaluation of movement, speech, sensation, and other specific functions of the nervous system. In some cases, an X-ray, CAT scan, or MRI scan of the brain can be helpful. Such an examination can help rule out head injury, stroke, tumors, or other lesions of the brain that could be responsible for cognitive changes.

Rule Out Head Injury or Stroke

A common cause of sudden decline in cognitive function is head injury. Many elderly people are unsteady on their feet, and it is not unusual for them to take a tumble and bump their heads. A little bump that is quickly shaken off should not be a major concern. However, if people who have taken a fall seem dazed or confused afterward, it is necessary to at least observe them carefully for several days. If they lose consciousness, even very briefly, or if you become suspicious about changes in their thought processes or behavior, it is important to get them to a doctor as soon as possible. The most serious concern is rupture of a small artery or vein in or around the brain. In elderly people with so-called hardening of the arteries, blood vessels can be fragile and tear easily. Moreover, when a person takes blood thinners such as warfarin for conditions such as atrial fibrillation or a history of blood clots, even a very small vessel losing blood can produce an ever-increasing pocket of blood inside the head that can cause changes in cognitive function or even threaten life itself. Over-the-counter medications, such as aspirin or ibuprofen, can also cause small injuries to bleed longer than they ordinarily would. Sudden changes in thought or behavior, with or without a witnessed incident of head injury, can also be the sign of a stroke. If suspicion is aroused, get to a doctor as soon as possible.

Rule Out Major Depression

A particularly important condition to rule out in patients suspected of having dementia is the so-called pseudodementia of major depression. Major depression is an illness that is often mistaken for dementia in elderly and even middle-aged patients. Major depression is at least as common among the elderly as it is among younger adults. In adults who are middle-aged, decreases in cognitive function are more likely to be due to major depression than to genuine, neurodegenerative dementia.

Not surprisingly, the elderly are more likely to suffer depression if they are disabled by health problems or if they are living in a nursing home instead of their own homes. Certainly, being older makes it more likely that an individual will have some type of disabling or activity-limiting form of illness. Nonetheless, among the otherwise healthy elderly living in their own homes, the rate of depression, about 2–4 percent, is no greater than that seen in other segments of the population.

To be certain of the diagnosis of dementia, major depression should first be ruled out. According to the DSM-IV, to make a diagnosis of major depression, it is necessary for a patient to exhibit two weeks of at least five of the following signs and symptoms of the illness:

- A depressed mood for most of the day.
- A lack of interest in or pleasure from activities the individual has previously enjoyed.
- A lack of appetite with weight loss, or, in some cases, an increase in appetite with weight gain.
- Insomnia or, in some cases, sleeping too much.
- Feeling exhausted most days.
- Moving and talking slowly, which is referred to as psychomotor retardation. In some people, there may be agitation and feelings of restlessness.

- Feelings of worthlessness, guilt, and remorse.
- Recurring thoughts of death and futility.
- Difficulty concentrating or indecisiveness.

There are no blood tests for diagnosing major depression. The diagnosis is entirely clinical. There are some standard sets of questions that can facilitate diagnosis of major depression. The Beck Depression Inventory, the Hamilton Rating Scale for Depression, and the Zung Self-Rating Depression Scale are three of the best-known tests that a doctor can perform in his or her office to help confirm the diagnosis of major depression. There is such a test designed for evaluating older patients called the Geriatric Depression Scale. However, all of these tests are similar in asking a variety of questions that address the nine basic diagnostic criteria for major depression that I noted above. In my experience, these tests are unlikely to reveal a case of depression that wasn't already suspected by simply talking with the patient and asking about his or her complaints. By and large, the diagnosis of major depression comes from the history given by the patient and from signs and symptoms that the patient and his or her family describe. Attentive and skillful clinicians should be able to determine if their patients meet the criteria for major depression as set out in the DSM-IV, but only if they bother to ask the appropriate questions.

There are some reports that depression is more likely to masquerade as vague aches and pains in elderly people than in younger patients. However, it is just as likely that physical complaints are under-recognized in younger adults with major depression. It is more likely among older adults to experience the grief of the loss of a spouse, siblings, or close friends who are also aging. Grief is a normal response, and it shouldn't be mistaken for the illness of major depression. However, in many ways it can resemble major depression, and if severe grief reactions continue for more than a few months, it is prudent to consider whether the grief response has evolved into an episode of major depression.

If a diagnosis of major depression is made, then treatment should be started without delay. After a few weeks for medication and/or psychotherapy to provide benefits, the MMSE and other evaluations of cognitive function should be repeated. In many cases, resolution of the major depression will also bring restoration of normal cognitive function.

Major depression in elderly people can be difficult to treat. Due to subtle differences in brain chemistry, or perhaps some decreases in the ability of medications to be taken up into brain tissue, medications that are helpful in young adults can be less than effective in people in their seventies or eighties. When the elderly do not respond to standard antidepressant treatments, it is prudent to seek the advice of a psychiatrist or a specialist in geriatric medicine. Of course, it must also be recognized that major depression and dementia can co-exist, and signs of dementia may remain independent of the mood disorder. In a later chapter I will discuss how a long personal history of major depression and other psychiatric illnesses can contribute to the development of dementia.

Rule Out Hormone and Vitamin Deficiencies

There are a number of laboratory tests that should be performed to rule out potentially reversible conditions that both contribute to major depression and mimic dementia. The most important tests are blood levels of vitamin B_{12}, the vitamin folic acid, and thyroid hormone. Vitamin B_{12} is essential for normal brain function, peripheral nerve activity, blood cell production, and other critical body functions. Vitamin B_{12} is a nutrient found only in food of animal origin, although it is also found in brewer's yeast. Vegetarians and other people with poor intake of foods containing B_{12} can suffer deficiency of this vitamin. In some cases, the intake of the vitamin is sufficient, but the body is unable to absorb the vitamin. Vitamin B_{12} deficiency is far more common than even most doctors realize it to be. Folic acid is another vitamin that acts as a biochemical partner of B_{12}. Folic acid deficiency, which is almost always the result of insufficient quantities of fruits, vegetables, eggs, organ meats, and other foods that contain the vitamin, can also contribute to cognitive dysfunction and mood disturbance. I more fully discuss vitamin B_{12} and folic acid deficiency as a cause of dementia in chapter 5.

Deficiency of thyroid hormone is a fairly common condition that should be ruled out in people who complain of feeling tired, low in mood, and slow in their thinking. The question I often ask my new patients who tell me they can't think clearly is if they feel their head is "full of bees" or "full of oatmeal." The "bees" answer is consistent with anxiety, attention deficit disorder, or bipolar affective disorder, whereas the "oatmeal" answer is consistent not only with major depression, but also a lack of thyroid hormone. Thyroid hormone levels are easily measured by a commonly performed blood test, and the condition is easily treated by supplementation with thyroid hormone in tablet form.

I feel obligated to note that while treatment of conditions such as thyroid hormone or vitamin deficiencies can sometimes reverse symptoms of dementia, in actual practice the results are often less than spectacular. In some cases the damage has already been done, and in other cases, the deficiency is only one of several pathological processes at work. Nonetheless, reversals and even cures of apparent dementias do occur, and it is wise to be vigilant and catch these deficiencies early.

Medications That Can Mimic Dementia

Another step that should be taken during the initial evaluation of suspected dementia is a thorough review of prescription and over-the-counter drugs the person may be taking. There are a number of such medications that can cause confusion and problems with memory and concentration. Many medications have a property called an anticholinergic effect. This refers to the ability of the drug to counteract the activity of a natural substance in the brain called acetylcholine. Acetylcholine is a major neurotransmitter, or chemical messenger that neurons use to communicate with each other. Most medications used to treat dementia act by increasing the activity of acetylcholine. Thus, it is not difficult to understand how a drug that blocks its activity could produce effects that might be mistaken for dementia.

Unfortunately, many of the maladies that older people suffer are treated with medications that have anticholinergic properties. One of the major anticholinergic culprits is the ordinarily quite benign substance diphenhydramine. Diphenhydramine is primarily used as an antihistamine for allergic reactions. However, since a major side effect of this non-addictive drug is drowsiness, it is frequently sold as an over-the-counter sleeping medication. It is a primary ingredient in the many of the so-called PM pain reliever preparations. I have frequently seen elderly people imprudently being given such medications to help them sleep when the aches and pains of arthritis and other ailments prevent them from getting the sleep they need.

Many older people, particularly women, may suffer urinary incontinence. Most of the medications used to treat this condition are strongly anticholinergic. An old type of antidepressant medication, the tricyclic antidepressants, has often been prescribed by doctors for complaints of pain and insomnia as well as for depressed mood. Such antidepressants, which include amitriptyline, imipramine, doxepine, and nortriptyline, have strong anticholinergic effects and are well known to cause confusion and memory problems in older patients. Medications for anxiety, such as valium and related substances, and the strong prescription opiate-based pain relievers, such as oxycodone, codeine, hydrocodone, and similar substances, can also cause confusion and cognitive disturbances that can be mistaken for dementia.

Delirium

Some medications and medical conditions can cause severe confusion, which is a condition referred to as delirium. Delirium is a dramatic disturbance in consciousness and awareness of the environment. It usually develops over a short period of time, and it not only causes problems with attention, language, and memory, but in severe cases may manifest in hallucinations and delusions. Delirious patients may act as if they are dreaming while awake. I vividly recall a patient I saw while I was still a medical student. He nearly scared me to death! Several days before he had undergone open heart surgery, and he was lying unconscious in the intensive care unit battling infections and other complications. As I stood by his bedside, he suddenly opened his eyes and began to scream, "Get out of my store!" He turned his eyes toward me, but looked right through me as if I were invisible. He grabbed an imaginary rifle and held it up to shoot in my direction, all the while yelling for me (or the "son of a bitch" he imagined was in his store) to get out or he would shoot. The seriousness of the disturbances in the chemistries of his body and brain was reflected in the fact that he died later that day.

Delirium can also be caused by too rapid a withdrawal of certain medications, particularly those used to treat anxiety and pain. The hallucinations and agitation of severe alcohol withdrawal, known as delirium tremens, is a well-known example of this condition. Other serious medical conditions, such as infections, electrolyte imbalances, low blood oxygen, liver failure, kidney disease, or hormone imbalances, can cause delirium. In some elderly people, simple urinary or respiratory infection can bring on delirium. Unfortunately, delirium is sometimes seen as merely the confusion of dementia, and it is not given proper attention. Because of the many serious and potentially life-threatening conditions that can cause delirium, any indication of delirium needs to be referred to a doctor as soon as possible.

SUPPORTING STUDIES: BRAIN SCANS AND TESTS OF BLOOD AND CEREBROSPINAL FLUID

A diagnosis of dementia is generally made when the behavior and function of a patient shows that he or she is not thinking well and this decrease in cognitive function isn't due to medical or psychiatric problems. More often than not, a careful review of the patient's history and the events that have led up to the concern about their behavior and function, as well as having ruled out medical or psychiatric problems as sources of these deficits, can be relied upon to provide an accurate diagnosis of dementia. However, in some cases, the presentation and history of a patient can be unusual or confusing to the doctor. When there is uncertainty about the diagnosis of dementia or about what type of dementia the patient is suffering, there are a number of more technical and, not surprisingly, more expensive tests that can be performed to solidify the diagnosis.

Although blood tests cannot diagnose Alzheimer's dementia, there are tests that can be performed to increase the likelihood that the clinical diagnosis of Alzheimer's is correct. For example, it is possible to use blood samples to determine what subtype of the APOE protein people have. APOE is a normal protein in the body that serves a number of important purposes. However, for reasons that are not entirely clear, inheriting the APOE4 variant of the protein is a major predisposing factor for developing Alzheimer's dementia. When changes in behavior and function that are consistent with Alzheimer's dementia are accompanied by the presence of the APOE4 protein, the evidence for Alzheimer's dementia becomes quite strong. It must be noted, however, that it is possible to have Alzheimer's dementia without the APOE4 protein, and, conversely, having the APOE4 protein does not guarantee that a person has or will develop this illness.

There are also tests that can be performed on cerebrospinal fluid to help confirm the diagnosis of neurodegenerative dementia. Cerebrospinal fluid, or CSF, is the fluid that bathes the brain and spinal cord. It cushions the brain and may also serve as a route of chemical communication and distribution of nutrients and other needed biochemicals. The unfortunate aspect of tests on CSF is that the fluid must be obtained by the procedure known as lumbar puncture or spinal tap. A needle is inserted between vertebrae in the lumbar or lower back region and guided into the pocket of CSF that surrounds the spinal cord. A small amount of fluid is drawn off and sent to the laboratory for analysis. Although it may sound rather dreadful, this procedure is done often during a day's work in a large hospital or emergency department, and it is simple and safe when performed by practiced hands.

In patients with Alzheimer's dementia, levels of tau protein are increased in CSF, whereas levels of amyloid are low, likely due to the fact that it is accumulating in brain tissue instead of being drained away and dispensed of by CSF. These changes can also be seen in many individuals who are in the very earliest stages of Alzheimer's dementia or in those with mild cognitive impairment. Thus, there are some advantages to going ahead with this invasive procedure. Other types of dementia, particularly Lewy body, frontotemporal, and vascular, can also generate higher levels of tau and lower levels of amyloid in CSF than would be expected in normal fluid samples. However, changes in Alzheimer's dementia are larger and more reliable for diagnosis. The presence of a brain protein known as 14-3-3 has been used to help diagnose Creutzfeldt-Jakob Disease (CJD), a rare neurodegenerative dementia that is often referred to as "mad cow disease" in the popular press. Curiously, amyloid levels tend to be high rather than low in the CSF of unfortunate patients with CJD.

AD7c is a protein that is contained in some neurons in the brain. It is significant because people with Alzheimer's dementia are often found to have higher levels of AD7c in their CSF. Thankfully, there are indications that levels of this protein are also high in the urine of patients with Alzheimer's dementia. Urine is lot more easily and painlessly obtained than CSF.

When changes in behavior and cognitive function are sudden or accompanied by neurological signs such as weakness of certain parts of the body, slurring of words, or loss of function of one side of the face or the body, high-tech brain scan methods are used to rule out things such as brain tumors, strokes, or infections. In some cases, these conditions can mimic the presentation of neurodegenerative dementia and need to be ruled out. On occasion, doctors want to rule out a relatively uncommon neurological disorder called normal pressure hydrocephalus (NPH), which can mimic dementia. NPH is a condition in which the structure of the brain is altered and function impaired by the buildup of fluid in chambers inside the brain known as ventricles. The three-part presentation of decreases in cognitive function, urinary incontinence, and unstable gait can sometimes lead an astute clinician to suspect NPH rather than one of the more common neurodegenerative forms of dementia. Telltale signs in a brain scan can help confirm the diagnosis of NPH. The distinction between NPH and neurodegenerative dementias is important because if caught in time and surgically treated, NPH can be reversed and cognitive function restored to normal.

Several different types of brain scans can be used to help confirm a diagnosis of dementia or to differentiate one type of dementia from another. A computerized axial tomography, or CAT, scan is the most commonly used form of brain scan. In most respects, a CAT scan is simply an X-ray of the brain. However, instead of a single snapshot, the CAT machine circles the head, sending X-rays through the tissue in such a manner that a computer can digitally reconstruct the brain in three dimensions. The computer can then project sections of the brain in fine detail either to film or a computer screen. Magnetic resonance imaging (MRI) provides much the same information as a CAT scan, but it is better able to spot areas of inflammation and compromised blood flow. Nonetheless, while these imaging techniques can help show that a change in behavior is the result of NPH, a hemorrhage, tumor, or other gross change in brain tissue, they can generally not be used to give a definitive diagnosis of any type of dementia, with the exception of vascular dementia. Indeed, many of the physical changes in the brain associated with dementia, such as shrinkage in brain size, can be found in many normal individuals, so obtaining such a finding proves little.

The sophisticated techniques of functional MRI, positron emission tomography (PET), and single photon emission computerized tomography (SPECT) can be used to visualize and measure the amount of metabolic activity in specific areas of the brain, and thus help determine exactly which areas are suffering from damage. These methods are often more reliable and informative than CAT or ordinary MRI scans in helping reach a diagnosis of dementia. However, they are quite expensive, and there is often a question as to how much more information they give beyond what an astute physician can gain from history, interviewing the patient and his or her family, physical examination, and neuropsychological testing. Still, there is a place for these techniques in dealing with difficult cases.

4

THE DEMENTIAS

According to the definition set out in the DSM-IV, the diagnosis of dementia requires that a patient exhibit disturbance in social or occupational function, as well as show deficits in memory and at least one of several other higher cognitive abilities. However, there are a number of different types of neurodegenerative illnesses that can cause dementia. The distinctions among the various types of dementia are important, because they can be quite different in terms of progression, prognosis, and treatment. Alzheimer's dementia is the most common form of this condition and, in the public mind, it has become synonymous with dementia. However, only about half of patients presenting with dementia are diagnosed as having Alzheimer's dementia. The next most common form of dementia is the vascular type, with about 30 percent of patients having this as the underlying cause of their dementia. Lewy body dementia is the next most common form and accounts for approximately 10 percent of cases of dementia. However, many experts believe that physicians often fail to recognize Lewy body dementia, and it is thus underdiagnosed and perhaps more common than previously suspected. Frontotemporal dementia is the least common of the major forms of dementia. There are also some rather rare forms of dementia, including Creutzfeldt-Jakob disease, AIDS-induced dementia, progressive supranuclear palsy, and Huntington's disease, which I will not further discuss.

MILD COGNITIVE IMPAIRMENT

Some patients present to their doctors with memory disturbance, yet without significant difficulties in judgment or deficits in their abilities to interact with their families, friends, and other social contacts. In the past, such a presentation has been referred to as age-related memory impairment. This is now more commonly referred to as mild cognitive impairment, or simply MCI. It is also becoming increasingly apparent that some individuals may retain memory function, but show signs of slight impairment of language or other higher functions of the mind. Moreover, whereas by definition MCI does not significantly disturb a person's social or occupational function, some individuals may have subtle difficulties in resolving social or work decisions that would have been easily resolved years before. Thus, the concept of MCI is evolving to include subtypes characterized by impairments of cognitive functions other than memory loss. These subtypes are referred to as non-amnestic MCIs. It is estimated that of seventy-year-olds who do not suffer dementia, roughly 5 percent do suffer MCI. This increases to 7 percent at age eighty.

There is a great deal of controversy as to whether MCI is a distinct illness, a mild form of dementia, or simply the early stages of an illness that will later manifest as a more obvious and severe dementia. Nonetheless, it has been found that over a year's time, about 15 percent of people with MCI will progress to meet criteria for diagnosis of dementia. In people with memory disturbance of an MCI level who also show evidence of other changes in cognitive function, such as personality changes, impaired judgment, or decreases in abstract thinking, the conversion rate to actual dementia is higher. Along with changes in cognitive function, about half of people diagnosed with MCI will also exhibit some form of mood disturbance such as depression, apathy, anxiety, or irritability. Because anxiety and depression can themselves adversely affect memory and other cognitive functions, a condition sometimes referred to as pseudodementia, it can sometimes be difficult to arrive at an accurate diagnosis early in the presentation of mood and cognitive disorders in people over the age of sixty.

ALZHEIMER'S DISEASE

Alzheimer's dementia was not the first type of dementia described in medical science. However, it is the most common and the most intensely studied form of dementia. The formal history of Alzheimer's dementia began in 1901, when Karl D. brought his fifty-one-year-old wife, Auguste D., to see the German neurologist Dr. Alois Alzheimer. Over a period of only a few years, she had developed problems with her memory and ability to perform her usual daily functions. She began to exhibit behaviors that were completely uncharacteristic of her usual way of acting. She had fits of anger and outbursts of screaming. She suffered hallucinations and delusions. She became insanely jealous of her husband and hid things about the house to protect them from people she suspected were out to steal them from her. Alzheimer could do nothing to help her, and she was eventually placed in an asylum. However, Alzheimer was so baffled by her precipitous decline that over the remaining five years of her life in the asylum, he continued to observe her and record his assessments. When she died, he removed her brain for study.

Alzheimer described Auguste D. in a lecture he delivered in 1906. However, the main portion of his observations was discussed in a publication by a colleague, Dr. Gaetano Perusini, in 1909, and it was primarily from that paper that we came to know Alzheimer's initial thoughts about his unfortunate patient and the nature of her illness. The original notes that Alzheimer took down during his examinations of Auguste D. were lost to science until they were rediscovered in Frankfurt, Germany, in 1995. The folder of patient records that was found in Frankfurt contained not only Alzheimer's notes of his observations of Auguste, but also several photographs of her. Although she was only fifty-six years old when she died, her appearance was one of a careworn, elderly woman, aged far beyond her years. An early excerpt from Alzheimer's notes reads: "She sits on the bed with a helpless expression. What is your name? *'Auguste.'* What is your husband's name? *'Auguste.'* Your husband? *'Ah, yes my husband.'* She looks as if she didn't understand the question. Are you married? *'To Auguste.'* Mrs. D? *'Yes, yes, Auguste D.'* . . . At lunch she eats cauliflower and pork. Asked what she is eating she answers, *'Spinach.'*" When Alzheimer asks her to write something, he records the following heart-wrenching episode: "When she has to write 'Mrs. Auguste D.,' she writes *"Mrs.,"* and we must repeat the other words because she forgets them. The patient is not able to progress in writing and repeats, *'Ich hab mich verloren'* (*'I have lost myself'*)."

The brain that Alzheimer removed from his patient was remarkably shrunken, and microscopic examination of it showed the tissue to be grossly abnormal. Alzheimer saw catastrophic loss of normal neurons and the presence of unusual plaques and tangles that had not previously been noted by neuropathologists. Although Alzheimer described the appearance of those plaques and tangles, he lacked the techniques needed to identify their chemical nature. Modern research has determined that the plaques are formed from what is essentially crystallization of an abnormal protein called amyloid. The tangles are knots of the protein tau, which is a substance normally found in neurons. Interestingly, the tissue samples that Alzheimer retrieved from Auguste D.'s brain in 1906 have also recently been rediscovered and studied by modern methods. Auguste D.'s brain was found to be free of any indications of vascular problems, stroke, or hardening of the arteries. There was, however, massive infiltration of amyloid plaques and neurofibrillary tangles of tau protein. Her brain gave evidence of a pure and perfect example of what has come to be referred to as Alzheimer's dementia.

Because of the relatively young age of Auguste D., and the rapid, precipitous decline she exhibited, it is likely that she suffered an extreme form of Alzheimer's disease. Her course of illness was not typical of most cases of the disease. Whereas her illness began in her late forties, the condition more commonly begins in a patient's late sixties. The illness as was first seen in Auguste D. is now referred to as the "early-onset" form of Alzheimer's dementia, whereas the form that manifests after the age of sixty-five is referred to as "late-onset" Alzheimer's dementia.

The convention of referring to these conditions as early-onset and late-onset forms of Alzheimer's dementia conveys the impression that they are simply two different manifestations of the same underlying pathology. Certainly, there are many similarities between these two conditions. Loss of memory is the primary sign in both conditions, and in both the substance of the brain is overwhelmed with plaques of amyloid protein and neurofibrillary tangles of hyperphosphorylated tau. However, there are reasons to believe that the so-called early- and late-onset forms of Alzheimer's dementia are two distinct illnesses. There are differences in the times of onset and courses of illness. There are also substantial differences in the frequencies in which these two types of dementia are seen to occur. Most significantly, there are substantial differences in the degree to which they are genetically determined and in which genes contribute to the characteristic damage to brain tissue.

In the case of Auguste D., symptoms of dementia appeared quite early in life, around the age of forty-nine or fifty. Her symptoms were quite severe by the age of fifty-one, which is when her husband brought her to see Dr. Alzheimer. This early emergence of severe dementia occurs in only about 5 percent of what are considered to be cases of Alzheimer's dementia. In most cases, symptoms of memory loss and decreases in the ability to function such that the patient meets criteria for diagnosis of dementia do not occur until after the age of sixty-five. Often, the signs and symptoms of dementia do not arise in individuals until they are in their seventies or eighties. In the unfortunate Auguste D.'s case, the dementia was also very rapid in progression, as is generally the case in early-onset forms of Alzheimer's dementia. In so-called late-onset Alzheimer's dementia, progression of the illness is slower. In most cases, the dementia is diagnosed in the moderately severe stage after years of subtle changes. It is generally two to four years after diagnosis that the illness progresses to the point that the individual requires some type of residential care. Unlike the precipitous decline of Auguste D., sufferers of late-onset Alzheimer's dementia often live another eight to twelve years after initial diagnosis. Many die of illnesses unrelated to dementia.

The most important distinction between early- and late-onset Alzheimer's dementia is the degree to which they are the result of genetic abnormalities. In almost all cases of early-onset Alzheimer's, at least one of three genes is found to be abnormal. These genes include the one that codes for amyloid precursor protein (APP), about which I will go into more detail later, and the genes that code for the proteins presenilin 1 and presenilin 2. The presenilin proteins are involved in the processing of APP. Errors in the DNA code can result in abnormal presenilin proteins that, in turn, increase the production of an abnormal sticky form of amyloid protein that accumulates in the brain as plaque. The only genetic abnormality that has been *consistently* associated with the late-onset form of Alzheimer's is the APOE4 gene. However, unlike the catastrophic abnormalities of the APP and presenilin genes, the mere presence of the APOE4 gene is neither necessary nor sufficient to cause Alzheimer's dementia. It simply makes the development of the illness more likely, its progression more rapid, and its manifestations more severe when other contributing factors are there. As I will explain later, these other factors are primarily those that emerge after unwise choices are made in matters of diet and lifestyle. Whether "late-onset Alzheimer's dementia" is a variation of the same illness Alzheimer first described in 1905 or something merely similar to that condition may be little more than an academic question. What is so very important is the fact that, unlike the majority of cases of the genetically predetermined early-onset form of Alzheimer's dementia, the late-onset form appears to be avoidable.

In cases of late-onset Alzheimer's dementia, the course of illness can vary from person to person. However, it is usually described as progressing in specific stages. I often conceptualize the progression of Alzheimer's and other forms of dementia as a shrinking of spheres of interaction with the world and one's own self. The first symptoms of Alzheimer's generally become apparent in dealings with the outside world. Above all, sufferers are forgetful. They have difficulty learning new things. Names of acquaintances are easily forgotten. They get behind in paying their bills. Checks bounce. They lose things and forget where the car is parked. The day comes when they get lost on the way to the market where they have driven hundreds of times before. It is quite common for anxiety and depression to evolve at this time. In some cases this can be due to the sufferer being aware enough to know that something is very wrong with them. In other cases, it is due to enduring the stresses of a life that has begun to unravel. This first stage of Alzheimer's dementia is generally thought to last two to three years.

As the disease progresses to the moderate stage, deficits begin to appear within the home sphere. Food rots in the refrigerator. Dishes pile up in the sink. The stove can be left on or food gets burned when food preparation is abandoned in midcourse. A person who was once meticulous in his or her habits may go days without bathing or wear clothes spotted with carelessly spilled food. As the moderate stage progresses, it is not unusual to see clothes put on inside out or briefs put on over, rather than under, a pair of pants. By this time, memory is very obviously deteriorating. Sufferers don't recall events that may have occurred earlier that day. Statements may be repeated, over and over.

My mother-in-law, who has always been, and to a surprising extent still remains, a charming, vivacious Southern belle, has been slowly drifting into a moderately severe stage of Alzheimer's dementia. She is now living in a residential care facility. We recently had her over for dinner, and large globe artichokes were on the menu. When my wife served the artichokes, her mother burst forth with glee and astonishment, "These are the biggest artichokes I have ever seen!" I then counted eleven more times during that relatively brief dinner that she again sang out with *exactly* the same lilting voice and *precisely* the same look of joy and surprise on her face that these were the biggest artichokes she had ever seen. On each occasion, she truly appeared to be seeing those artichokes for the very first time.[1] It has often mistakenly been suggested by people naïve to the disorder that Alzheimer's and other forms of dementia are simply reversions to childhood patterns of behavior. Such a notion was dispelled when my nine-year-old son finally said with a mild sense of annoyance, "Why do you keep saying that?"

---

1. This is an example of the maintenance of semantic memory but failure of episodic memory that is common in Alzheimer's dementia. She recognized the appearance of an inordinately large artichoke, which is in the realm of semantic memory, but failed to recall through episodic memory that she had already expressed her amazement at the size of the artichokes on the table in front of her. It is also an example of the deficit in retaining information as new memories.

In moderately severe Alzheimer's dementia it becomes more difficult to find words for common objects, and names of even close friends or relatives might be forgotten. In fortunate cases, the patient may experience a slide into serene befuddlement. However, severe anxiety or outbursts of anger can occur. It is not uncommon for sufferers to begin to imagine things. They might imagine that a favorite bowl they mistakenly threw in the trash was stolen by neighbors. A common suspicion is that family members are conspiring to control them or to take away their house or savings.

A fairly common and puzzling phenomenon that may emerge at this time is an increase in confusion and agitation in the early evening. This is often referred to as "sundowning." Sundowning is estimated to occur in about 15 percent of individuals with Alzheimer's dementia. However, it is not unique to this form of dementia, as it also is seen in vascular, Lewy body, and frontotemporal dementias. This recurring emergence of confusion as night falls has been explained in many different ways. It most cases it reflects a larger disturbance in circadian rhythm that is part of the neurodegenerative process of dementia. Individuals with sundowning also tend to have sleep irregularities during the night. It has been suggested that sundowning is the result of dream states emerging into consciousness. Another explanation has been that the frontal cortex, which processes and understands information about the world, falls asleep, while the lower, more primitive activating systems of the brain continue to keep other areas of the cortex awake and active. It is possible that these disturbances are due to degeneration of the suprachiasmatic nucleus of the brain, which is seen by neurobiologists as the location of the brain's internal timekeeping mechanism. It has also been noted that sundowning may reflect a disturbance in hormone levels, particularly that of melatonin. Supplementing with melatonin has been reported to improve both sleep abnormalities and sundowning behaviors. Interestingly, the APP23 strain of mice, which are genetically engineered to develop an Alzheimer's-like condition, show disturbances in the sleep-wake cycle that are reminiscent of the circadian disturbances in humans with Alzheimer's dementia.

It is in the moderate stage that families begin to wonder about their loved one's ability to function at home. They may begin to consider assisted living or nursing home placement. Episodes of violence or fecal incontinence are often the "last straws" that lead a family to arrange such placement. The moderate stage of Alzheimer's tends to last another three to four years.

In the final stage of Alzheimer's, which stretches over the last three to four years of life, cognitive functions continue to deteriorate. Whereas in the moderate stage a sufferer may wear clothes spotted with spilled food, in more advanced stages simply putting on clothes becomes an impossible task. Patients may be oriented to self, but they lose conception of time and place. Even spouses and children may no longer be recognized. In time, patients forget their own names as well. Delusions and emotional outbursts can be fueled by delirium and hallucinations. Eventually the illness reaches a stage where control of the body itself is lost. This is the dreadful stage 7 of the Global Deterioration Scale, in which "the brain appears to no longer be able to tell the body what to do." Speech deteriorates and patients have great difficulty expressing themselves. Sufferers generally become incontinent of bladder and bowels. They are unable to feed themselves. Walking becomes more difficult, and a point is reached when patients become bedbound or must be restrained to prevent falls. Alzheimer's itself does not kill, but death often comes from combinations of weakness, dehydration, failure to eat, and pneumonia. The pneumonia is often the result of aspiration of food or fluid and inability to guard the airway and generate an adequate cough reflex.

VASCULAR DEMENTIA

Vascular Dementia is a form of dementia that arises when blood flow to the brain has been compromised by cardiovascular disease, that is, disease of the heart and blood vessels. This compromise can be a reduction in blood flow, with resulting poor function of neurons due to lack of adequate oxygen and fuel, or a complete loss of blood flow, with resulting death of affected areas of brain tissue. The complete loss of blood flow to an area of the brain is commonly called a stroke. A stroke can result either from a blockage of an artery in the brain by a clot, which is referred to as an embolic stroke, or from the bursting of an artery in the brain, which is called a hemorrhagic stroke. Sometimes a "preview of coming events" may be experienced when an artery is temporarily blocked by a clot but later becomes open again when enzymes in the blood are able to dissolve the clot. The temporary loss and regaining of function is called a transient ischemic attack, or TIA. TIAs serve as warning signs of permanent losses of function that may occur if proper steps aren't taken to treat the underlying problems.

After Alzheimer's dementia, vascular dementia is the second most common cause of dementia. However, because many individuals with Alzheimer's and other forms of dementia also suffer cardiovascular disease, it is not uncommon for those patients to suffer vascular dementia as well. This form of illness is referred to as mixed dementia. It is thought that 20 percent or more of people with Alzheimer's dementia in fact suffer a mixed dementia. However, there are reasons to suspect that 20 percent is an underestimation.

One reason for the common occurrence of mixed dementia is that dietary and other lifestyle choices that increase the risk for cardiovascular disease also increase the risk of developing Alzheimer's dementia and, quite likely, Lewy body and frontotemporal dementias as well. Vascular dementia also compounds the damage from the other forms of neurodegenerative dementia. Although loss of blood supply can cause direct and rapid loss of cognitive function, damage to blood vessels in the brain can also more indirectly stimulate the progression of the other types of dementia by triggering pathological processes such as inflammation, stress responses, and leakage of membranes that ordinarily protect the brain from harmful substances in the blood. Despite the fact that oxygen supply to the brain decreases with reduction of blood flow, oxidative damage may actually increase when brain tissue is chronically deprived of adequate blood supply. This seemingly paradoxical effect comes about because damaged cells have a reduced ability to protect themselves from the toxic effects of reactive substances produced in the use of oxygen to burn fuel.

There are several different subtypes of vascular dementia. The most obvious kind is the sudden and dramatic loss of cognitive function that can follow a major stroke. The effects of a stroke are entirely dependent upon what area of the brain is deprived of its blood supply. Some areas of the brain are more involved with movement and sensation than they are with cognitive functions. While a stroke may cause significant loss of movement and dexterity, it is estimated that less than 30 percent of strokes result in vascular dementia, as defined by a loss of cognitive function that interferes with social interaction, work, and activities of daily living. Unfortunately, it is not uncommon for the conditions that caused the first stroke to persist and produce subsequent strokes over time. If the series of strokes affects areas of the brain more obviously involved in cognitive function, this can result in what is referred to as multi-infarct dementia. Infarct is the medical term for the death of tissue in a specific area after it has been cut off from its blood supply.

One of the hallmarks of multi-infarct dementia is a stepwise loss of cognitive function. Stepwise loss is in contrast with the gradual but steady loss of function that is common in Alzheimer's dementia. For example, a patient with relatively normal cognitive function may suddenly begin to have difficulty naming objects. This symptom may persist without further change for months or more, until a sudden change in usual behavior appears in addition to the inability to name objects. Other aspects of cognitive and, not uncommonly, motor and sensory functions may then begin to be lost in sudden, serial fashion. Another manifestation of multi-infarct dementia is significant losses of some mental functions, but surprisingly good retention of others. I sometimes describe this phenomenon to patients and families as the "Swiss cheese effect," with "holes" appearing here and there in otherwise normal areas of cognitive function.

Understandably, a stroke can cause substantial anxiety and depression, particularly if loss of speech and motor function make it difficult to communicate, alter facial appearance, or rob patients of their ability to participate in favorite activities. It is estimated that 25 to 50 percent of patients may experience an episode of major depression after suffering a stroke. Since major depression itself can cause difficulty with memory and concentration, a reversible condition called pseudodementia, the degree of loss of cognitive function from the stroke itself may sometimes be difficult to assess. It should also be noted that strokes in certain areas of the brain can cause abnormal expressions of emotion. For example, a patient may speak in a loud, whining, tearful manner even while denying feeling particularly sad or depressed at that moment. This phenomenon is called pseudobulbar affect. It can be very disturbing to witness, but thankfully it is often temporary.

Although strokes can cause sudden and dramatic loss of cognitive function, some vascular problems can produce more gradual loss of function, more like what is seen in Alzheimer's dementia. In 1894, Dr. Otto Binswanger described a condition of cognitive decline often accompanied by difficulty walking and urinary incontinence. Sometimes, the sufferer can experience seizures. This type of vascular dementia tends to emerge around the age of sixty, after years of high blood pressure and hardening of the arteries, or what doctors refer to as arteriosclerosis. Damage to the sensitive inner walls of small arteries that serve the brain reduces their ability to carry oxygen and fuel into brain tissue. This results in oxidative stress, inflammation, and diminished function of neurons. Tissue damage is most often seen in white matter lying in subcortical areas of the brain. Unlike gray matter, which contains cell bodies of neurons, white matter contains the transmission lines that connect neurons across different parts of the brain. When these lines are damaged, the "command and control" systems of the mind and body break down. Binswanger called the illness he described in 1894 "encephalitis subcorticalis chronica progressiva." In 1902, Alzheimer referred to it as Binswanger's disease, which remained its name for most of the twentieth century. This type of vascular dementia is now referred to as subcortical ischemic dementia (SCID).

A rarer form of SCID is an illness called cerebral autosomal dominant arteriopathy with subcortical infarctions and leukoencephalopathy, mercifully abbreviated as CADASIL. In CADASIL, individuals are born with abnormalities in the small blood vessels of the brain, which eventually result in decrease of blood flow and actual tissue loss in areas of white matter. Signs and symptoms of the disease include migraine headaches and depression, as well as losses of cognitive function. In this illness, symptoms may begin in patients who are still quite young, sometimes emerging in their forties or fifties. There is thought to be about one case of CADASIL per fifty thousand people. However, it may be underrecognized.

LEWY BODY DEMENTIA

Lewy bodies are microscopic protein deposits in brain cells that were named after Dr. Friedrich Heinrich Lewy, a German-born neurologist who was a colleague of Dr. Alzheimer's. Lewy first described these bodies in 1912 after observing them in the brains of patients with Parkinson's disease. In patients with that illness, the Lewy bodies were most prevalent in an area of the brain called the substantia nigra. The substantia nigra is populated by neurons that produce and release the neurotransmitter dopamine, and the presence of Lewy bodies in these neurons has contributed to our recognition of the fact that loss of dopamine-producing cells in the brain is primarily responsible for the motor deficits seen in Parkinson's disease. The reason that Lewy bodies are so prominent in neurons that produce dopamine is that the metabolism of dopamine involves oxidative processes that make the cell vulnerable to oxidative damage. When damage is limited to dopamine-producing cells, the result is Parkinson's disease. It is not clear why cells other than dopamine-producing cells can become vulnerable to Lewy body formation, or if oxidative damage plays a role in that pathology.

In 1923, Lewy further reported that these bodies could sometimes also be found in areas of the brain where the higher functions of mind originate. He noted that many individuals who had these Lewy bodies in their cerebral cortex exhibited evidence of dementia. It is unfortunate that this finding of Lewy's languished for over fifty years before it was recognized that the presence of Lewy bodies in the cerebral cortex defined a unique and surprisingly common form of dementia that is now referred to as Lewy body dementia. Although the numbers are not clearly known, it is suspected that after Alzheimer's dementia, Lewy body dementia might eventually be recognized as the second most likely cause of dementia in older adults.

As with Alzheimer's dementia, the basis for a suspicion of Lewy body dementia lies in the observation of changes in cognitive function that interfere with the individual's performance of their activities of daily living. In many respects, the signs and symptoms of Lewy body dementia are similar to those of Alzheimer's dementia. Signs that are generally considered to help distinguish Lewy body from Alzheimer's disease include slightly less loss of memory in the early stages of Lewy body dementia, fluctuations in severity of symptoms, the presence of visual hallucinations, and motor symptoms suggestive of Parkinson's disease.

Patients with Alzheimer's dementia can have good and bad days. However, even on good days, the basic problems with memory and judgment persist, and there is rarely any doubt that the patient is suffering a persistent and progressive loss of cognitive function. In contrast, patients with Lewy body dementia, particularly when symptoms are first presenting, can exhibit striking lapses in memory, judgment, and attention, but only days later seem to be their same old selves again. Visual hallucinations can occur in Alzheimer's patients, particularly in the later stages. However, the visual hallucinations that are frequently described by patients with Lewy body dementia can be quite extraordinary. I recall a patient I was evaluating who suddenly, yet very politely, asked for a pause in our conversation so that he could watch the horses that were galloping down the hallway. Patients with Lewy body dementia may be prone to such vivid and complex visual hallucinations because the degenerative processes in the illness tend to quickly spread to the posterior, occipital areas of the cortex that process visual information. This is less often the case in Alzheimer's dementia.

The medical literature is less clear about the average age of onset of Lewy body dementia than it is with Alzheimer's dementia. This may be because up until recently, Lewy body dementia has been poorly recognized and thus diagnosed relatively late in the course of illness. Nonetheless, there is little reason to suspect that the age of appearance of symptoms of Lewy body dementia is any different from that of Alzheimer's. This has certainly been the case in my experience.

Lewy body dementia is clearly related to Parkinson's disease, and the appearance of Lewy bodies in neurons is the hallmark of both conditions. However, Lewy body formation can begin in different areas of the brain, with resulting differences in manifestations and presentation. Although Lewy body dementia will sometimes be diagnosed in patients who have already been diagnosed with Parkinson's disease, it can also manifest in patients who do not exhibit the classical signs and symptoms of Parkinson's. For example, the so-called pill rolling tremor that so often characterizes

Parkinson's disease is not always seen in Lewy body dementia. Nonetheless, after cognitive changes, visual hallucinations, and fluctuations in severity of symptoms, the fourth most common diagnostic sign of Lewy body dementia is frequent falling. For years before the widespread recognition of Lewy body dementia as a specific illness, neurologists had described a form of dementia that not infrequently developed in the later stages of Parkinson's disease. However, many neurologists and psychiatrists believe that this so-called Parkinson's dementia and Lewy body dementia are one and the same condition.

The Lewy bodies that define Lewy body dementia are formed from aberrant collections of a brain protein called synuclein. Synuclein can collect in abnormal knots of protein in a manner similar to the way that amyloid precursor protein crystallizes into plaques in the brains of patients with Alzheimer's disease. One of the risk factors for Lewy body dementia is a family history of the illness, which suggests a genetic predisposition to develop the condition. This may be due to inheritance of abnormal variant forms of synuclein, or abnormalities in the enzymes that process the protein. However, as has been found to be the case in Alzheimer's dementia, pathological processes such as oxidation, inflammation, and high cholesterol accelerate the abnormal laying down of synuclein in brain tissue. Thus, unhealthy dietary and other lifestyle choices may exacerbate conditions that cause pathological deposition of synuclein, amyloid, and tau protein. This may explain why many patients with Lewy body dementia are later found to also have the amyloid plaques and neurofibrillary tangles that characterize Alzheimer's dementia. Of course, there is no basis to assume that an unfortunate individual couldn't suffer from both Alzheimer's and Lewy body dementia. In fact, pure cases of one type of dementia versus another may be the exception rather than the rule.

A condition sometimes seen in the elderly that is characterized by visual hallucinations, and which can thus easily be mistaken for Lewy body dementia, is Charles Bonnet syndrome. This fascinating syndrome gets its name from the Swiss naturalist and philosopher Charles Bonnet. In 1760, Bonnet described reports of cognitively healthy elderly people seeing visions of people, birds, horses, buildings, geometric patterns, and other complex visions. The person experiencing these visions is almost always aware that these visions are not real. Nonetheless, the hallucinations are extremely realistic and compelling.

Charles Bonnet syndrome occurs primarily in elderly people who have begun to lose their sight, either due to eye problems such as macular degeneration or after vascular problems or strokes have damaged visual pathways in their brains. It is usually short lived and generally lasts no more than a few years. Most neurologists suspect that these visions are similar to the strange hallucinations reported by people in sensory deprivation tanks. When the brain is deprived of its usual sensory information, in this case through disturbances in the visual system, it starts to simply invent things. The mind is then left to try its best to make sense of it.

A peculiar aspect of these hallucinations is that the people in the visions are often "Lilliputian," that is, it is not uncommon for them to be seen as little people in costumes. I vividly recall an elderly woman in her early nineties who was brought to my office by her family when they were concerned about her reports of seeing "little men" in her living room. At first she was quick to explain that she knew these men were not real. However, over time she began to lose the capacity to convince herself that these extremely realistic visions were simply manifestations of her aging eyes and brain. I suspect that she was beginning to develop some dementia along with the Charles Bonnet syndrome she had at first exhibited. In any case, it wasn't too many months before she began to spray these little men with an aerosol can of insecticide. I recall with certain affection for her that she vehemently denied being afraid of them; rather she insisted she was simply annoyed at them for sitting in her house but refusing to answer her questions. She felt they were being intolerably rude.

Another patient of mine was also in her nineties when she began to see compelling visions of people outside of her home. I believe that her visions were due to poor blood supply to the visual processing centers in the back of her brain. This woman remained well aware of the fact that these people were a product of her own mind. The hallucinations were certainly not the result of dementia. In fact, what was so remarkable about her was how extremely well preserved her overall cognitive function continued to be throughout the time I saw her. Although she visited my office only every two weeks, she was able to repeat in fine detail what we had discussed in the previous session. She was always completely oriented to time and place and was well versed in current events. She had a wonderful sense of humor, and I found her to be very pleasant company. She never showed the slightest indication of suffering dementia.

Aside from providing some comfort in explaining to her and her family why she was experiencing the hallucinations, there was really little else I had to offer her. After three or four visits, I discharged her from my care. I understand she remained stable until a few months later, when some other medical problems arose. Those problems sapped her vitality and led to her death.

PICK'S DISEASE AND FRONTOTEMPORAL DEMENTIA

In 1892, fifteen years before Alzheimer's report about his female patient with severe and rapidly progressing dementia, the Czechoslovakian neurologist and psychiatrist Arnold Pick described what appeared to be a new form of dementia characterized by marked atrophy of the frontal and temporal lobes of the brain. Patients who at autopsy were found to have this atrophy had often lost their ability to speak or appeared completely unmotivated to communicate. They also had behavioral abnormalities, such as apathy, social withdrawal, lack of empathy for other people, and inattention. Curiously, some patients behaved in quite the opposite fashion, showing impulsivity, inappropriate displays of strong emotions, a tendency to disrobe in public, or excessive familiarity with strangers. Despite what could be dramatic changes in language and behavior, there was usually relatively little loss of memory in the early stages.

The apathy and withdrawal of these patients can be similar to what is seen in major depression, whereas the disinhibited, inappropriate behaviors can resemble those seen in mania. Thus, it is sometimes first suspected that the individual is suffering a psychiatric disorder rather than dementia. Accurate diagnosis is further complicated by the cruel fact that the disease can appear in people as early as their forties or fifties, which is often thought to be too young to have a dementing illness.

More than thirty years after Pick's report, peculiar spots that the discoverers called Pick bodies were found in brain tissue of patients with the dementia and behavioral changes that he had described in 1892. However, researchers were puzzled by the fact that these Pick bodies, which were later found to contain tau protein, occurred in only a small percentage of these patients. The early techniques did not reveal that most patients suffering Pick's disease have small bodies in their brains that contain a different protein called ubiquitin. At one time, Pick's disease was thought to be a rare condition. However, it is now believed that Pick's disease represents a spectrum of closely related degenerative brain disorders, some with classical Pick bodies, but most with ubiquitin-containing bodies alone, which together account for 10 percent or more of cases of dementia.

Whereas the lesions of Alzheimer's dementia are seen primarily in the parietal and posterior temporal lobes of the brain, in Pick's disease, changes are noted primarily in the frontal and anterior temporal lobes. This has led to the replacement of the name Pick's disease with the term frontotemporal lobar dementia, or FTLD. Most neuroscientists believe that it is our highly developed frontal lobes that most clearly differentiate us from other primates and give us our uniquely human qualities. It is the frontal lobes that give us "personhood." They are extremely complicated areas of the brain and control a variety of critical cognitive functions. The neighboring temporal lobes contribute to functions of memory, as well as those of language and speech. Along with the loss of cognitive function that defines dementia, frontotemporal dementia is characterized by various combinations of apathy, loss of inhibitions, or impulsivity; lack of insight; poverty of speech, decreased emotion, and decreased empathy; violation of social and moral norms; changes in eating behavior; and repetitive behaviors.

The design of the frontal lobes is complicated, to the point that parts of these lobes that are immediately adjacent to each other can be responsible for quite different aspects of cognitive function. For this reason, neuroscientists have come to recognize several different subtypes of frontotemporal dementia that differ from one another by exactly where in the frontal lobes the neurodegenerative processes begin and what symptoms predominate in the patient's presentation. Degeneration of the orbitobasal areas of the frontal lobes, which rest just above and behind the eyes, tends to result in impulsivity and loss of social inhibitions. Damage to the medial areas, which lie behind the middle of the forehead, leaves the individual apathetic and unmotivated to move or speak. Loss of function of the dorsolateral areas, which rest behind the sides of the forehead, disrupts attention, logic, planning, judgment, and mental flexibility. Sufferers of dorsolateral frontal lobe dementia lack insight, develop narrow preoccupations, or repeat senseless activities. When the degenerative processes affect the temporal lobes, either as the first signs or as a subsequent stage of the illness, speech becomes affected. Speech can become nonsensical in content or gradually decrease in amount and in the level of its complexity. Unlike Alzheimer's dementia, in which memory loss is the primary and invariable finding, memory disturbance in early stages of frontotemporal dementia is variable. In the later stages of the illness, memory loss is virtually certain to occur.

In many cases, a person with frontotemporal dementia can experience and exhibit all of these different symptoms in a progressive fashion as the degenerative process works its way through the frontal and temporal lobes. This is certainly the way in which my father experienced this dreadful illness. Initially, he began to show peculiar yet subtle changes in his social behavior. I recall one telling incident in which a family reunion brought relatives from all across the country to meet in Kansas City. We were together in a banquet hall of a hotel where we enjoyed dinner together. After our meal, members of our rather large extended family came to the microphone at the front of the hall to speak a few, or not so few, words about how wonderful it was to be all together again. After several others had offered their comments, one of our cousins rose from his seat and lumbered over to the microphone. This particular cousin could kindly be described as "odd." However, as a member of the family, his eccentricity in manner, obesity, and ill-fitting clothes were always given some allowance. As our cousin stood before us and fumbled with the paper upon which he had written his speech, my father let loose with a loud, prolonged, and heartfelt "Oh, my God!" Although most of us were thinking precisely the same thing, my father's outburst broke the rules of social engagement and gave embarrassing testimony to the early stage of his illness.

Over the next few years, my father had increasing difficulty expressing himself. His word choices sometimes made no sense. A sad but undeniably humorous example arose when a couple my parents knew invited them to tour the prestigious Nelson Gallery of Art in Kansas City. This big, beautiful old gallery is built of stone, with high ceilings and long hallways. Please excuse the indelicacy, as I must relate that in quite unrestrained fashion, my father passed gas loudly and forcefully in one of the exhibition rooms, and the report echoed down the spacious corridors. That lapse in social grace was simply another product of the insidious process of frontal lobe degeneration. However, for days afterward he perseverated in reporting his troubling perception that their friends were very angry with him "because I *fluctuated* at the art gallery." Even when challenged about his choice of the word "fluctuated," he simply looked puzzled and then continued on using the word to express his annoyance with himself and his friends.

Gradually, my father drifted into apathy and a complete inability to speak at all. Not too many months after he lost speech, his final indignity was to suffer the loss of his ability to swallow. That unfortunate man, who so dearly loved a good meal, was thus deprived of his last pleasure. Eventually a tube was inserted through his abdomen and into his stomach to provide him nourishment. The last time I saw my father, he was propped up in a chair staring impassively, neither moving nor speaking. He turned his eyes toward my face and let them linger for the briefest of moments, which served as the only evidence of any recognition of who I was. Not many months later, he died in his sleep, which I am sure was a blessing for him.

BEYOND ALZHEIMER'S

In the public mind, Alzheimer's and dementia are virtually one and the same. It is also commonly believed that if one of your parents has suffered dementia, then you too are destined to develop the same condition. Neither of these perceptions is true. It is important to get beyond these simple notions about dementia to be able to prevent and treat modern occurrences of this condition.

Alzheimer's disease is only one of several different types of neurodegenerative diseases that present with loss of cognitive function. Alzheimer's accounts for just under half of reported cases of dementia, with Lewy body, vascular, and frontotemporal dementias making up the majority of the remaining cases. "Pure" forms of these different types of dementias can be seen in some patients. Such distinctions can be important, as courses of illness can differ, and certain medications can more useful for one versus another type of dementia. However, more often than not, patients present with forms of dementia that are mixed in the types of behaviors and cognitive losses that can be observed, as well as in the pathological changes that occur in their brains.

Some forms of dementia are quite clearly genetic, and thus are forms that can be inherited from one's parents. The classical, early-onset form of Alzheimer's dementia, such as arose in the unfortunate Auguste D. in her early fifties, is almost certainly genetic in basis, as are the early-onset forms of frontotemporal, Lewy body, and vascular dementias. If you inherit these genes, then you are quite likely to develop the dementia and to do so at a relatively young age. However, the illness first described by Alzheimer just over one hundred years ago is not typical of the forms of dementia being seen today. In fact, the cases of dementia that are currently appearing in people in their late sixties and early seventies are often not the classical forms of any specific type of dementia. Although some dementias do begin as distinct classical forms, the distinguishing features of specific types of dementia tend to grow indistinct as the conditions progress in each patient. My father, for example, exhibited many signs and symptoms consistent with classical frontotemporal dementia. However, he did not begin to exhibit his symptoms until he was in his mid sixties, which is a little later in life than is typically seen in classical forms of the illness. My father also suffered from high cholesterol, high blood pressure, and coronary artery disease. Along with some components of vascular dementia, he also likely suffered some subtle brain damage from the bypass surgery he underwent in his early sixties.

Medical researchers have begun to note that in so-called sporadic cases of dementia, regardless of the type, there appear to be similar underlying pathological conditions that trigger the start and progression of the illness. While certain genes may predispose the bearer to specific presentations of dementia, those genes do not necessarily cause the illness. For most people, it may be more accurate and useful to go beyond Alzheimer's, frontotemporal, Lewy body, or vascular dementias to see most modern dementias as somewhat different presentations of several basic neurodegenerative processes fueled by poor diet, insulin resistance, metabolic syndrome, stress, inflammation, poor sleep, lack of mental and physical stimulation, poor habits, environmental toxins, and other effects of ill-chosen ways of living.

5

WHAT CAUSES DEMENTIA?

GENETICS

Some people are genetically predisposed to develop dementia. It has long been recognized that the early-onset form of Alzheimer's dementia, in which loss of cognitive function is evident before the age of sixty-five, runs in families and has a strong genetic basis. However, the early-onset form accounts for only about 5 percent of Alzheimer's cases. The majority of cases of Alzheimer's dementia are diagnosed after the age of sixty-five in people for whom there is no strong family history of the illness. This more common presentation is called sporadic Alzheimer's dementia.

One of the best ways to evaluate the degree to which an illness is genetically determined is to compare the incidence of the illness among sets of identical and fraternal twins. Several studies on the development of sporadic, late-onset Alzheimer's dementia in twins have been performed. It has been found that identical twins are nearly twice as likely as fraternal twins to both suffer Alzheimer's dementia. Because identical twins share exactly the same genetic information, but fraternal twins do not, these findings show that the risk of developing the common late-onset form of Alzheimer's is influenced by genetics. However, it is critical to note that late-onset Alzheimer's dementia is seen in both identical twins only about half of the time.[1] Thus, it must further be concluded that genetic factors do not guarantee that a person will develop the illness. The current belief among researchers is that genes increase the risk of Alzheimer's dementia, but certain adverse environmental and lifestyle factors are likely to be necessary for the illness to begin and progress.

A number of genes have been identified as contributing to Alzheimer's dementia. In the relatively rare, early-onset forms of the disease, there are usually genes that produce abnormal forms of amyloid precursor protein or the enzymes that process that protein. Two genes that code for proteins involved in processing amyloid, presenilin 1 and presenilin 2, are often found to be abnormal in patients with early-onset Alzheimer's dementia. It is not yet clear if, diagnosed early enough, those individuals with seriously abnormal genes can avoid dementia.

A gene variant that contributes to both the early-onset and sporadic forms of Alzheimer's is the E4 subtype of apolipoprotein E, which is more commonly referred to as APOE4. APOE is a normal and necessary protein in the brain. Among the functions of the APOE protein are controlling the amount of amyloid precursor protein that gets produced and helping the brain to rid itself of the 1-42 fragments that form the abnormal beta amyloid. APOE4 does not perform this function as well as the other forms of the protein, and thus it predisposes its owners to the accumulation of beta amyloid in the brain. If people inherit two copies of the E4 subtype, that is, one copy from each parent, then they are more likely to develop the abnormal plaques of amyloid protein that characterize Alzheimer's dementia and to develop them at an early age. There are tests that can be performed to determine which subtypes of APOE people carry and whether or not an APOE4 gene places them at increased risk of dementia. However, finding one or even two copies of APOE4 does not serve as a positive diagnostic test for Alzheimer's dementia, nor does it guarantee that the individual will at any time develop the illness. Given the fact that APOE4 is neither necessary nor sufficient to cause Alzheimer's dementia, one can only conclude that its primary adverse effect is to amplify and aggravate other factors that disturb the complex chemistry of APP and amyloid protein processing in the brain. In fact, the APOE4 gene not only increases the risk of Alzheimer's dementia, but also increases the risk of cardiovascular disease and vascular dementia by increasing bad (low-

---

1. You must realize that in growing up together, identical twins tend develop similar tastes in food and predilections for lifestyles that may influence risk for developing dementia. Although these risks are shared, they are not genetic in nature. They may also share genetic predispositions to heart disease, diabetes, or other factors that only indirectly affect risk for dementia.

density lipoprotein, or LDL) cholesterol, triglycerides, inflammation, and oxidative damage.

More is known about the genetics of Alzheimer's dementia than about the other major forms of neurodegenerative dementia. However, as with Alzheimer's, there are known to be early-onset forms of those dementias that are almost certainly genetically determined. These early forms probably reflect abnormalities of genes that code for proteins that collect as abnormal deposits in the brain tissue of sufferers of the illnesses. In the case of frontotemporal dementia, these are the proteins tau and ubiquitin, and in Lewy body dementia, this is the protein synuclein. As with Alzheimer's, most cases of frontotemporal and Lewy body dementias are of the sporadic type. It is possible that certain genes predispose people to develop the sporadic forms of the illnesses. However, as with Alzheimer's dementia, these genes probably only increase the risk and do not necessarily cause the diseases. Again, it is likely that environmental and lifestyle factors are required for these illnesses to manifest.

With the rare exception of CADASIL, there are no gene abnormalities that directly produce vascular dementia. Rather, the risk of vascular dementia goes up in people who carry the APOE4 gene and those who are otherwise genetically at risk for heart disease, high blood pressure, high LDL cholesterol, diabetes, and other medical conditions that damage the walls and linings of small blood vessels in the brain and throughout the body. Certainly, there are some unfortunate families that carry genes that increase their risk for developing those cardiovascular conditions. However, in most people, this risk is a function of poor diet, lack of exercise, high levels of stress, and other factors more closely related to bad choices than bad genes. Thus, while some people may be genetically predisposed to vascular dementia, in most people this form of dementia can be avoided.

Neurodegenerative dementias fall across a wide spectrum in terms of the degree to which they are the result of genes inherited from parents. On one end of the spectrum are the severe, early-onset forms of dementia that are the virtually inevitable result of the presence of specific genetic abnormalities. On the other end of this spectrum are cases of dementia that occur in people who have no obvious genetic predisposition to dementia, but have subjected their bodies to the adverse effects of unhealthy lifestyle choices. In between are dementias in which certain genes may predispose the individual to dementia, but those genes are neither necessary nor sufficient to produce the dementia. Those dementias arise because of poor diet, unhealthy lifestyle choices, and environmental factors, with genes merely making dementia more likely and helping to determine what the characteristics of the dementia will be once the process of neurodegeneration has begun.

AMYLOID PLAQUES AND PROTEIN TANGLES

Alzheimer's dementia, the most common form of neurodegenerative disease, is characterized by the presence of amyloid plaques and neurofibrillary tangles of tau protein in the brain tissue. These plaques and tangles are also seen to some extent in the brains of patients with other types of dementia, and even in the brains of elderly people who retain normal cognitive function. What are amyloid and tau proteins, and how do they contribute to dementia?

The term amyloid does not refer to a specific protein, nor to abnormalities of proteins that are unique to the brain. In fact, many different types of amyloids can occur in tissues of the body. Amyloids are the result of abnormal processes that can turn a variety of harmless, naturally occurring proteins in the body into unruly, sticky masses of crystallized protein that begin to build up where they don't belong. For example, the devastating illness called amyloidosis is caused by accumulations of proteins that originate from cells of the immune system. Although this abnormal form of protein can be deposited in the brain, in patients suffering amyloidosis it more typically gets lodged in the heart, lungs, and other organs.

The specific protein that accumulates as abnormal amyloid plaque in the brains of patients with Alzheimer's dementia is referred to as amyloid precursor protein, or APP. It is not entirely certain what role APP plays in normal brain function. However, APP is known to be essential. Eliminating all of the genes that code for APP in mouse brains, a genetic engineering procedure known as creating the APP "knock-out" mouse, is lethal for those animals.

Most proteins in the body are first produced as long chains of amino acids, which are later sliced by enzymes at specific points to release a perfectly tailored protein segment from the chain. Different segments from the original larger chain can often have different roles in body chemistry. Whereas the segment of APP that stretches from amino acids 1 to 40 is harmless, the segment of amino acids 1 to 42 is sticky and difficult to get rid of once it is formed. Segment 1-42 is the protein that crystallizes into amyloid plaque. A number of different problems can increase the likelihood that the sticky segment 1-42 of APP is produced in the brain. In some cases, a person can inherit a variant form of APP that is more likely to be cleaved between amino acids 42 and 43 and thus is predisposed to generating more sticky 1-42 segments of protein. This is known to be the basis for some inherited forms of early-onset Alzheimer's dementia. Another cause of genetic predisposition to Alzheimer's dementia is the inheritance of enzymes that tend to splice normal APP into 1-42 segments. In other cases, aptly named "chaperone" proteins that escort 1-42 segments out of the brain don't perform their job properly. Some 1-42 APP segments are always produced, even in normal brains, and the lack of effective chaperone proteins allows this form of APP to build up.

Amyloid from APP is what accumulates in Alzheimer's dementia. However, other types of amyloid characterize the other forms of neurodegenerative dementia. The protein synuclein can accumulate as amyloid in Lewy body dementia, and ubiquitin amyloid may gather in certain frontotemporal dementias. It is likely that problems in processing, splicing, and disposal of abnormal protein segments, analogous to those I described for amyloid deposition in Alzheimer's dementia, are responsible for accumulation of abnormal protein in these conditions as well.

Although abnormalities in handling of protein in the various forms of dementia can be inherited, many such abnormalities arise out of poor lifestyle choices. It is known, for example, that insulin resistance, stress, lack of important nutrients, oxidative damage, and inflammation can cause the activity of otherwise normal APP, splicing enzymes, and chaperone proteins to go awry. This results in the over-production and accumulation of sticky, plaque-producing 1-42 amyloid in the brain. The accumulation of amyloid itself can stimulate inflammatory responses as part of the brain's attempt to rid itself of the abnormal protein. The protein structure of amyloid may also interfere with the actions of insulin and increase insulin resistance in brain tissue. The accumulation of amyloid thus participates in an upward spiral of damage to tissue, including accelerating further buildup of yet more amyloid.

Tau is another natural protein in the brain. Tau is largely a scaffolding protein that helps to form what is often referred to as the microskeletons of neurons in the brain. The microskeleton gives shape to neurons and provides structures to anchor systems of transport within them. As is quite often the case in cell biology, the addition of what is called a phosphate group acts like an on-or-off switch for proteins, and this is the case with tau. Tau that does not have phosphate groups attached to it cannot interact with the protein of the microtubules that carry needed substances back and forth across the cell. However, if tau is given too many phosphate groups, that is, if it becomes what scientists call hyperphosphorylated, serious problems begin to happen in the neuron. One problem that can occur is that hyperphosphorylated tau becomes sticky and can clog up important pore-like channels in the membrane that encloses the neuron. This interferes with transmission of chemical signals between neurons, and it can cause "noise" in the communication among neurons in the brain. Disruption by hyper-phosphorylated tau of the activity of a particular channel called the NMDA receptor can contribute to dementia. This particular disruption occurs not only in Alzheimer's dementia, but also in the dementia that can result from HIV infection of the brain. The disruption of NMDA receptor activity in Alzheimer's and HIV/AIDS dementias can both be treated with the drug memantine, which physicians can prescribe for dementia.

Another problem that can result from hyperphosphorylation of tau is that the tau protein fibers stick together and form knots of protein called neurofibrillary tangles. These big knots of protein interfere with normal cell processes, and they may eventually trigger the process of apoptosis, or programmed cellular suicide. Neurofibrillary tangles are characteristic of Alzheimer's and several other types of dementia. Hyperphosphorylation of tau is quite common in frontotemporal dementia.

A number of abnormalities can cause hyperphosphorylation of tau. Some individuals are genetically predisposed to it. However, as is the case with deposition of amyloid plaques in the brain, a wide variety of problems that tend to arise from poor lifestyle choices can increase the risk of hyperphos-phorylation. Among the problems that can stimulate hyperphosphorylation are the stress hormone cortisol, inflammation, damage from oxidation and free radicals, and the insulin resistance that evolves in metabolic syndrome.

METABOLIC SYNDROME

Among the primary risk factors for dementia are heart disease and diabe-tes. In many, if not most, cases those conditions arise in people who have failed to control metabolic syndrome. This condition is becoming increas-ing common in our country and in developed countries around the world. It is estimated that up to 30 percent of the adult population in the United States could be diagnosed as having metabolic syndrome, and this percent-age increases to over 40 percent of people over the age of sixty. Not only adults, but also children are at risk for developing metabolic syndrome. A recent and sobering study has shown that roughly 16 percent of children and adolescents in the United States are obese. Of those obese children, as many as 30 percent show signs of metabolic syndrome.

A syndrome is a constellation of problems that on the surface seem unrelated, but in fact are all due to a single underlying cause. Metabolic syndrome manifests as a combination of high blood pressure, high fasting glucose levels, high levels of fat in the form of triglycerides in the blood, low levels of good (high-density lipoprotein, or HDL) cholesterol, and abdominal obesity. Dr. Gerald Reaven, the Stanford physician and researcher who discovered metabolic syndrome, found that these seemingly unrelated signs are all the result of the body becoming increasingly resistant to the hormone insulin.

Reaven initially recognized that the high blood pressure and LDL cholesterol levels of metabolic syndrome led to heart disease, whereas the high serum glucose and the stress this placed on the pancreas eventually led to diabetes. However, since he first formally described the syndrome in 1988, he came to realize that along with those illnesses, the insulin resistance that lies at the bottom of metabolic syndrome also predisposes people to conditions as various as gout, sleep apnea, polycystic ovaries, and even certain forms of cancer. It has become increasingly clear that metabolic syndrome and its underlying insulin resistance also increase a person's risk of developing dementia.

Let me explain why insulin is so very important in the body. In humans and other animals, the main type of sugar carried in the blood is glucose. Glucose and fat are the main sources of energy in the body. A high level of glucose, such as might occur after eating a meal rich in carbohydrates, stimulates the pancreas to produce and release insulin, whose main job is to reduce those levels of glucose in the blood. Insulin reduces blood glucose by acting on liver, muscle, and fat cells. Between meals, when blood glucose levels start to drop, the liver is able to produce glucose and release it into the blood to maintain an adequate supply. After a meal, when the body has all the glucose it needs, insulin tells the liver to stop releasing glucose into the blood and, instead, to take up glucose from the blood and store it for future use in the form of the starch-like molecule glycogen. The liver also converts extra calories from carbohydrate into saturated fat, which is another process stimulated by insulin. Insulin then further stimulates the liver to release this fat, in the form of triglyceride bound in cholesterol, into the blood for delivery to fat cells for storage. Muscle cells are stimulated by insulin to more efficiently take up glucose from the blood and use it for fuel. By stimulating fat cells to take up fat from the blood, insulin further reduces blood glucose by forcing the muscle cells to use glucose rather than the fat they actually prefer as fuel. These various effects of insulin act in concert not only to reduce blood glucose levels, but to shift the body from fasting state to nourished state. Extra calories can then be stored away for future use, while still maintaining an adequate supply of fuel for the body.

The importance of insulin to the body is seen in the fact that prior to the discovery of insulin, children with juvenile diabetes, who were unable to produce their own insulin, invariably died of their illness. In metabolic syndrome, people do not lack insulin; rather their bodies become less responsive or resistant to the effects of this critical hormone. It is not entirely clear what causes insulin resistance and, in turn, metabolic syndrome. Some unfortunate individuals are born with a genetic tendency toward insulin resistance. However, most often it is genetic predisposition in combination with indiscretions of diet and lifestyle that lead to metabolic syndrome. Generally, this is a matter of too much sugar and saturated fat, too little exercise, too little sleep, and lots of stress.

One of the clues that first led Reaven to discover metabolic syndrome was a study by Dr. Edward Ahrens performed in the early 1960s at The Rockefeller University in New York City. Ahrens had found that most people with high concentrations of fat in the form of triglycerides in their blood acquired that condition not from eating too much fat, but rather from eating too much carbohydrate. This counterintuitive finding arises from the fact that many people are simply unable to safely utilize large amounts of carbohydrate consumed on a regular basis. Some of these individuals have a genetically low sensitivity to insulin, and a steady diet high in carbohydrate requires the pancreas to continually pump out large amounts of insulin to bring glucose levels back to normal level. This constant exposure to high concentrations of insulin helps set the processes of metabolic syndrome into motion. Even in people who are not genetically predisposed to insulin resistance, unhealthy diet and lifestyle eventually wear away at natural sensitivity to insulin and bring about insulin resistance and metabolic syndrome. When scientists want to study metabolic syndrome in laboratory animals, they produce this syndrome in otherwise healthy animals simply by feeding them large amounts of sugar.

The irony of metabolic syndrome is that the body suffers not only from lack of insulin's effects in resistant tissue, but also from the abnormally high levels of insulin that are then required to maintain normal blood glucose levels. This paradoxical situation arises out of the fact that the decreases in response to insulin can progress at different rates in different tissues throughout the body. Even in any one organ, some responses to insulin may remain intact while others will show resistance. For example, whereas the liver grows resistant to insulin's signal to stop churning out glucose, the organ remains sensitive to insulin's command to package fat in packets of cholesterol and release it out into the blood to be picked up by fat cells for storage. The consumption of large amounts of rapidly absorbed carbohydrates in this state leads to the high glucose along with high triglyceride and cholesterol in the blood that largely defines metabolic syndrome.

Metabolic syndrome is a progressive illness. When the body is over-whelmed with sugar and saturated fat, either from the diet or from the fat produced by the liver out of the extra carbohydrate, subtle damage begins to appear in cells throughout the body. Fat collects deep within cells where it doesn't belong, such as in and around the mitochondria. Unlike fat cells, liver and muscle cells aren't designed to hold this dangerous substance, and it begins to disrupt cellular functions. Similarly, too much sugar flood-ing the body interferes with the usual safe handling of this fuel. Reactive molecules called free radicals and abnormal combination of glucose with proteins, or glycation, can result. Those pathological processes in turn trig-ger inflammatory reactions and stress responses. The damage caused by the poor control of glucose and fat only increases the underlying resistance to insulin in tissues throughout the body, and this causes the problem to spiral further out of control.

Medical researchers have discovered over the past twenty years or so that fat cells play a surprisingly important role both in the progression of meta-bolic syndrome and in the damage that the syndrome can cause in tissues throughout the body. Although fat cells, or adipocytes, used to be thought of as simple warehouses of fat, they are in fact extremely complex cells with the extraordinarily important job of monitoring the body's storage and utilization of a very dangerous fuel. A particularly important population of fat cells resides in the abdominal cavity and are referred to as visceral adi-pocytes. The visceral adipocytes orchestrate the distribution and handling of fat throughout the body by releasing hormones called adipocytokines. When the visceral fat cells become overburdened with stored fat, they lose their usual fine control of the release of the adipocytokines. When excreted in excess, some adipocytokines can cause further resistance to insulin, as well as inflammation, changes in appetite, and other abnormalities that fuel the progression of metabolic syndrome.

All of the changes that define metabolic syndrome, that is, the high blood pressure, increases in blood sugar, and high levels of fat and bad cholesterol in the blood, increase the likelihood of dementia. The high blood pressure damages fine blood vessels in the brain, and if severe and persistent enough, can lead to Binswanger's form of vascular dementia. Inflamed blood vessels in the presence of high levels of fat lead to atherosclerosis, blood clots, strokes, and multi-infarct dementia. Poorly controlled glucose and fat metabolism leads to oxidative stress in brain tissue, which accelerates the neurodegen-erative processes that underlie Alzheimer's, Lewy body, and frontotemporal dementias. Abnormal levels of adipocytokines released by visceral fat cells adversely affect the brain by triggering inflammation and other abnormal processes. In what has come as something of a surprise to neuroscientists, it appears that insulin resistance in the brain itself may be a major contributor to neurodegeneration and the development of dementia.

METABOLIC SYNDROME, THE BRAIN, AND DEMENTIA

The brain's primary fuel is glucose. However, unlike muscle cells, the brain does not depend on the action of insulin to enhance its uptake of glucose. In fact, for many years, scientists thought that, aside from acting in the ancient and primitive part of the brain called the hypothalamus to regulate appetite and calorie intake, insulin had no important effects on the primary functions of the brain. Therefore, the scientific world was surprised in 1967 when high concentrations of insulin were found in cerebrospinal fluid, which is the fluid that bathes and cushions the brain. In 1978, insulin receptors were identified in the brain, not only in areas of the brain that help control appetite, but even in areas involved in higher brain functions, including memory. If insulin wasn't necessary for neurons to take up glucose for fuel, then what was it doing in the brain?

There are now a number of studies showing that insulin acts in the brain to help maintain cognitive function. Injection of insulin directly into the brains of rats has been found to improve certain types of learning. On the other hand, injection of streptozotocin, a substance that disrupts insulin signaling in the brain, causes long-term and progressive losses of cognitive function in those animals. Several studies using human subjects have similarly shown that increasing insulin activity in the brain can improve cognitive function.

Intravenous or subcutaneous administration of insulin can be extraordinarily dangerous. It can cause blood glucose to drop to potentially lethal low levels. In one laboratory study, this danger was avoided by giving insulin intravenously along with exactly the right amount of glucose necessary to maintain normal blood glucose levels. Subjects who received the extra insulin showed significant improvement in memory and other tests of cognitive function. In a similar study, in which Alzheimer's patients and a control group were administered insulin and glucose in that fashion, the subjects with dementia showed improvement in verbal memory. Curiously, the insulin improved the cognitive function of the patients with Alzheimer's dementia more than it did for the normal control subjects.

Administration of insulin up the nostrils in a nasal spray has also been found to enhance memory in human subjects. Apparently, insulin can enter the olfactory nerves that carry information about odors and travel up these nerves to enter the brain itself. In fact, the hippocampus, which is an area of the brain critical for the laying down of new memories, is immediately adjacent to the areas of the brain that process the sense of smell.[2] Intranasal administration of insulin did not significantly alter blood levels of glucose; thus it may be both a safe and convenient means to increase levels of insulin in brain tissue to improve or at least maintain cognitive performance. However, this is an experimental and risky procedure, and certainly *not* something to try at home!

Although resistance to insulin in the liver, muscles, and adipocytes is what is most clearly associated with metabolic syndrome, it has been found that under these circumstances, the brain also begins to be less responsive to insulin. Insulin resistance, in both rodents and human beings, is associated with decline in cognitive function. In one interesting study, mice genetically altered to produce human brain proteins were made insulin-resistant by feeding them large amounts of sugar in their diet. In fundamental respects, their condition resembled metabolic syndrome in humans. It was then revealed that the learning ability of these animals was impaired. Moreover, their brains were found to have increases in the numbers of amyloid plaques, such as is found in the brains of humans with Alzheimer's dementia. Other studies have shown that learning and memory are improved in animal models of Alzheimer's after treatment with insulin. Thus it appears that insulin can enhance cognitive function, whereas disturbance in insulin activity, such as is found in metabolic syndrome, can disrupt it.

Insulin affects cognitive function and risk of dementia in part through affecting the processing of amyloid in the brain. A study presented to the International Conference on Alzheimer's Disease in 2008 showed that people with diabetes who take both insulin and drugs called oral hypoglycemics, which enhance the effects of insulin, can have lower burdens of amyloid than even those who do not suffer diabetes. One way in which insulin controls amyloid accumulation in the brain is by limiting production and release of amyloid precursor protein, from which beta amyloid is made.

---

2. In Marcel Proust's famous book *Swan's Way*, the first in the series that makes up *Remembrance of Things Past*, he describes how as an adult, the smell of Madeline cakes dipped in lime blossom tea evoked full and exquisitely detailed memories from his childhood. This phenomenon has come to be referred to as "Proustian memory," and it likely arises from the fact that memory and the processing of the sense of smell are inextricably bound in the structural evolution of the brain and, hence, the mind.

Another way that insulin decreases amyloid deposition is by stimulating the production of insulin degrading enzyme, or IDE. As you might expect, this is the same enzyme the body uses to rid itself of insulin after the hormone has does its job. When evolution has supplied the body with a useful and effective enzyme, such as IDE, it is not so unusual for such an enzyme to perform multiple tasks in the body. It so happens that amyloid and insulin have enough structural similarities that IDE can also act to destroy amyloid that it comes in contact with. The brain knows how much IDE to produce by sensing how much insulin is in the tissue. Thus, when tissue is resistant to insulin, not enough IDE is produced. There is then less IDE to gobble up not only insulin, but the abnormal deposits of amyloid as well. The final insult is that the structural similarities between amyloid and insulin allow amyloid to interact with insulin receptors in the brain and block the activity of insulin. Thus amyloid, in effect, further increases insulin resistance in the brain.

Along with affecting amyloid, insulin has also been found to affect the processing of tau, the protein in the brain that forms neurofibrillary tangles in the brains of patients with Alzheimer's dementia. In studies of mice genetically engineered to have defective insulin receptors in their brains, the processing of tau protein becomes abnormal in ways very similar to what is seen in brains of Alzheimer's patients. Tau becomes hyperphosphorylated, forms tangles, and causes cellular dysfunction and death.

Insulin also helps prevent degeneration of brain tissue and dementia by limiting the activity of an enzyme called glycogen synthase kinase-3beta, or GSK-3. GSK-3 is an ancient enzyme that is found in every cell of the body. In the liver, GSK-3 prevents the storage of glucose in the starch-like substance glycogen. Blocking glycogen production increases the amount of glucose in the liver and makes it more available for release into the blood. Insulin inhibits GSK-3, thereby stimulating the storage of glucose in the form of glycogen. This decreases blood glucose levels, which is the primary goal of insulin release.

GSK-3 is also found in the brain and, as in the liver and other tissues in the body, insulin acts in brain cells to inhibit the activity of GSK-3. The brain does not produce or store glycogen, thus the ability of GSK-3 to inhibit glycogen synthesis has no relevance in the brain. However, there are many important effects of GSK-3 that are of significance in the development of dementia. Among the effects of GSK-3 are stimulation of amyloid precursor protein production and phosphorylation of tau protein. The neurofibrillary tangles that are seen in both Alzheimer's and frontotemporal dementias are due to hyperphosphorylation of tau protein. When insulin is prevented from inhibiting GSK-3 because of the resistance to insulin that occurs in metabolic syndrome, the processes of amyloid deposition and hyperphosphorylation of tau both increase. GSK-3 also stimulates nuclear factor-kappaB (NF-κB), which is one of the important triggers of inflammation in the brain and other tissues. A lack of insulin activity increases inflammatory processes in the brain that go on to exacerbate neurodegeneration. In fact, recent studies have found that insulin has anti-inflammatory effects, which may be due, in part, to inhibition of GSK-3 activity. Finally, it has been found that GSK-3 stimulates the process of apoptosis, which is genetically programmed cell death. Inhibition of GSK-3 by insulin and other substances increases the number of neurons in the hippocampus of the brain in part by turning off apoptosis.

THE "THIN" HORMONE, LEPTIN

Recently it has become clear that the hormone leptin, one of the adipocytokines released from visceral fat cells, is involved in metabolic syndrome, appetite control, mood modulation, and maintenance of cognitive function. There is growing evidence that deficits in leptin activity in the brain contribute to neurodegeneration and dementia. Leptin was discovered in 1994 after scientists began to pursue the question of why a particular strain of laboratory mouse was prone to developing obesity. It turned out that this mouse, known to scientists as the *ob/ob* mouse, lacked a gene to produce a specific protein.[3] When this protein was administered to those deficient mice, their voracious appetites for food decreased, they lost weight, and they returned to a normal size. The protein was called leptin, which is derived from the Greek work for thin.

For a time there was great excitement in the scientific community over the possibility that the evasive "thin" gene had finally been identified. Doctors assumed that, like the *ob/ob* mouse, obese humans might be lacking in the ability to produce adequate amounts of leptin. They hoped that by administering leptin to their obese patients, they would be able to restore normal appetite and allow them to reach a normal, healthy weight. A revolution in weight control seemed to be at hand. However, much to the surprise and disappointment of scientists, the vast majority of obese humans were found not to be deficient in levels of leptin in their blood. In fact, reminiscent of

---

3. The term *ob/ob* simply refers to both of the mouse's inherited leptin genes being defective, which leads to *ob*-esity in these animals.

the hyperinsulinemia seen in metabolic syndrome, these obese subjects were generally found to have abnormally *high* blood levels of leptin.

Leptin is produced primarily in fat cells, and it was soon learned that the amount of fat stored within an individual fat cell determines how much leptin that cell produces and excretes into the bloodstream. The reason people with obesity have such high levels of leptin is simply because they have so much fat being stored in their bodies. Since leptin controlled appetite and weight in *ob/ob* mice, and obese people had high levels of leptin in their blood, focus shifted to the question of how the body might lose its ability to respond to leptin's command to stop eating.

A great deal has been learned over the past ten years about the phenomenon of leptin resistance. For example, it has been learned that some of the same problems that cause obesity may also interfere with the effects of leptin. High levels of fat, particularly saturated fat, in the diet can alter the chemistry of neurons in the hypothalamus of the brain where leptin acts to control appetite. Too much fructose in the diet can also disturb cellular response to leptin. Leptin resistance is frequently seen as a component of metabolic syndrome. The high levels of triglycerides and other forms of fat in the blood that occur in metabolic syndrome may cause the same changes in the hypothalamus that are seen with high dietary fat. The compensatory increases in the blood levels of insulin that occur in metabolic syndrome may contribute to diminished responses to leptin in the body. There is even evidence that high levels of leptin may interfere with its own activity. In some respects, this resembles the tolerance that develops with other chemical messengers or in cases where medications have been used at high doses for a long period of time.

Although resistance to leptin may play a role in the failure of leptin to control appetite in the obese, there is also evidence that leptin may not get into the brain in sufficient quantity in these individuals. Even though obese people may have high levels of leptin in their blood, the ratio of leptin in their brains versus in their blood is relatively low in comparison to what is observed in lean individuals. High levels of fat in the diet, and hence in the blood, can prevent leptin from crossing the blood-brain barrier, which separates and buffers the brain from substances in the bloodstream. The high levels of triglycerides seen in metabolic syndrome can cause the same effect.

Increases in serum levels of C-reactive protein (CRP), which is released into the blood in various inflammatory states, including metabolic syndrome, may also reduce levels of leptin in the brain. Apparently, CRP can bind to leptin and thus prevent it from being taken up from the blood and transported into the brain. Ovariectomized rats, which exhibit the same loss of estrogen as occurs in menopausal women, do not appear to transport leptin into their brains as well as females with normal estrogen levels. Aging also appears to reduce the efficiency with which leptin is transported into the brain.

In studies using obese but otherwise normal rats, injection of leptin into the body had no effect on their appetite or weight. In view of the fact that these animals already had high levels of leptin in their blood, it came as no surprise that adding more leptin to their blood had no effect on their food intake. Nonetheless, administration of leptin directly into their brains did reduce their appetite and lead them to lose weight. Thus, while resistance to leptin can and does occur in the brain, it may be less of a problem than leptin resistance in the rest of the body. This would allow the possibility of development of medications that could mimic the effects of leptin but more easily pass through the blood-brain barrier into the hypothalamus to control appetite. Administering leptin directly into the brain is effective in laboratory animals, but obviously infeasible in human patients. However, as with insulin, there are animal studies suggesting that intranasal administration of leptin can increase brain levels of leptin and effectively reduce appetite and weight in leptin-deficient animals. To the best of my knowledge, there have not yet been such studies in humans.

Leptin affects appetite by acting in the hypothalamus. As was the case with insulin, neuroscientists at first saw leptin as having no other important effects in the brain. They certainly had no reason to suspect that this hormone produced in fat cells could possibly have effects in areas of the brain involved in higher functions of the mind. However, leptin receptors have recently been found to exist not only in the hypothalamus, but throughout the brain, including in the cortex, where higher cognitive processing takes place. Laboratory rats and mice that are genetically deficient in leptin perform poorly in tests of learning and memory. The process of long-term potentiation (LTP), a neural process essential for learning, is disturbed in the hippocampus of these animals. Administration of leptin directly into their brains restored normal LTP and improved learning and memory. Deficiencies in leptin activity have also recently been associated with mood changes, and it is thought that leptin may play a role in mood disorders such as major depression. There is even evidence that leptin, like insulin, may be produced in certain areas of the brain itself to help maintain normal function.

Current evidence further indicates that leptin may serve an important neuroprotective function in the brain. Leptin reduces the production of amyloid protein in the brain and helps mobilize abnormal forms of the protein for more rapid removal from brain tissue. In mice that have been genetically engineered to develop the same type of amyloid plaques found in patients with Alzheimer's dementia, chronic treatment with leptin decreased the amount of amyloid deposited in brain tissue. Leptin has also been found to prevent the hyperphosphorylation of tau protein that leads to the neurofibrillary tangles in Alzheimer's and other neurodegenerative diseases. Leptin blocks the cellular suicide pathway of apoptosis in neurons and is protective of neurons in states of stress and low oxygen.

Together, the data suggest that leptin can increase rates of survival of neurons after acute insults such as strokes or during chronic neurodegenerative changes such as are found in Alzheimer's dementia, Parkinson's disease, and other neurological disorders. Conversely, a lack of leptin, or possibly leptin resistance, in the brain may contribute to cell death and the progression of dementia. In both demented and normal aged individuals, the amount of gray matter in the hippocampus and adjacent areas of the cortex has been found to vary directly with blood levels of leptin. Interestingly, in patients with Alzheimer's dementia, leptin levels in the blood tend to be low.

DIABETES

Diabetes is an illness that presents as a persistent state of high blood sugar. Diabetes is diagnosed when a fasting blood glucose level is found to be higher than 126 mg/ml. This increased level of glucose is due to one of two reasons: either the body doesn't produce enough insulin or it no longer responds to this critically important hormone.

Diabetes in its classical form, which is now called diabetes type 1, occurs when the body's response to insulin is normal, but the pancreas is damaged and unable to secrete a sufficient amount of insulin. This form of diabetes usually develops before the age of thirty, and it is not uncommon for it to begin in childhood. That condition has been referred to as juvenile-onset diabetes, and it affects as many as one out of every thousand children. Diabetes type 1 is often caused by autoimmune disease, in which the body's immune system is somehow triggered to attack cells in the pancreas that produce insulin. Only about 10 percent of cases of diabetes are type 1.

The more common form of diabetes, which is referred to as diabetes type 2, is caused by the body no longer being able to respond to insulin. Diabetes type 2 tends to occur in adults and, not surprisingly, it generally evolves out of metabolic syndrome. The same poor choices in diet, high levels of stress, lack of exercise, and insufficient sleep that lead to metabolic syndrome also lead to diabetes type 2. An ominous report from the U.S. Centers for Disease Control and Prevention in 2008 states that in the past ten years, reports of new cases of diabetes type 2 have doubled.

Diabetes is quite often associated with high blood pressure, high cholesterol, heart disease, and stroke. According to the American Diabetes Association, about 65 percent of people with diabetes die from heart disease or stroke. A lot of the damage seen in the bodies of people with diabetes is caused by the abnormalities of metabolic syndrome, which begin before blood sugar levels become high enough to be diagnosed as diabetes. Unfortunately, the onset of diabetes does not end the ongoing process of metabolic syndrome. High bad cholesterol, high triglycerides, and hypertension tend to persist unless aggressively treated. Moreover, obtaining insulin by injection, rather than through release from the pancreas, does not improve the body's sensitivity to it. It is often the case that, reminiscent of the pancreas increasing its output of insulin to keep up with resistance, people with diabetes often have to gradually increase their dose of insulin to maintain the same levels of blood glucose, due to continued increases in insulin resistance.

Although much of the damage of diabetes is from the problems that began as metabolic syndrome, it is fair and accurate to say that everything that metabolic syndrome does that is bad for the body, diabetes only makes worse. The high blood glucose levels that distinguish diabetes from metabolic syndrome are particularly damaging to the body and the brain. When cells are flooded with glucose, the mitochondria can lose control of some of the dangerous side products of the glucose oxidation process. The most dangerous side product is the oxygen free radical. This type of free radical is an oxygen atom that has been given an extra electron, and it cannot wait to unload it on any unsuspecting molecule that happens to be nearby. This oxidative damage, and the toll this process takes on the body, is referred to as oxidative stress. Cellular structures are damaged and inflammatory processes are stimulated by free radicals.

Too much glucose also results in proteins having glucose chemically bonded to their molecular structures, which results in loss of activity and inability of the cell to rid itself of the products. These protein and sugar aggregates, called advanced glycation endproducts (AGEs) also stimulate further inflammatory reactions. Although Alzheimer's dementia is most strongly associated with accumulations of amyloid and tau protein, high blood glucose causes the addition of abnormal chains of glucose derivatives to the plaques and tangles in the tissue of the brain, which appears to accelerate the degenerative process.

High blood glucose can, in the short term, cause confusion and slowness in thought processing. In the long run it increases the risk of Alzheimer's dementia. Because of the damage that occurs in small arteries in the brain, it also increases the risk of the multi-infarct and Binswanger's forms of vascular dementia through stroke, hypertension, and subcortical ischemia. In young patients with type 1 diabetes who have suffered this illness for fifteen to twenty-five years, decreases in gray matter in the brain, indicating decreases in the number and size of neurons, have been observed. The reduction in volume of their gray matter appeared to be a reflection of how high their blood glucose had been over the years. A new study, published in the journal *Neuropsychology*, has now conclusively shown what has long been suspected: individuals with diagnoses of diabetes type 2, even those as young as their early fifties, show deficits in cognitive function compared to age-matched individuals without diabetes. Such deficits can occur even among patients considered to have relatively mild diabetes type 2.

LOW BLOOD SUGAR

A different abnormality of glucose level that is sometimes seen in diabetics is low blood glucose, or what physicians refer to as hypoglycemia. Hypoglycemia can occur in diabetics when administration of insulin or other medicines to lower blood glucose overshoots the goal of normalizing glucose and causes blood glucose to plummet to dangerously low levels. Alternating episodes of high and low blood glucose are thought to cause serious damage to the brain and hasten the development of dementia.

Although high carbohydrate diets contribute to high blood glucose, metabolic syndrome, and diabetes, meals high in easily digested carbohydrates can also produce post-prandial or "after eating" hypoglycemia. Foods that have a high glycemic index, that is, foods that quickly raise blood glucose after they are consumed, can stimulate large and sudden bursts of insulin from the pancreas. In susceptible people, this burst of insulin can cause a too-rapid decline in blood glucose. If blood glucose falls below 60 mg/ml, then symptoms of anxiety, sweating, mood changes, and confusion can result.[4] This can be par-

---

4. The notion that hypoglycemia is a major cause of psychiatric illness was popularized by the endocrinologist Dr. Emmanuel Abrahamson in his 1951 book, *Body, Mind, and Sugar*. Abrahamson stated, "Hypoglycemia might be the physical background to the portrait of the so-called neurotic in all or at least in the vast majority of cases." Post-prandial hypoglycemia can certainly contribute to major depression, anxiety, and other psychiatric conditions. However, research over the past fifty years has shown that post-prandial hypoglycemia being the primary cause of psychiatric illness is by far the exception rather than the rule.

ticularly serious when compromise in liver or adrenal gland function prevents the body from quickly raising serum glucose levels back to normal. Episodes of post-prandial hypoglycemia may also be more likely among individuals whose pancreatic function has been compromised by metabolic syndrome. This phenomenon is sometimes referred to as dysinsulinemia.

The hippocampal area of the brain is particularly sensitive to lack of glucose for fuel, and hypoglycemia interferes with memory and cognitive processing. Hypoglycemia causes severe oxidative stress in neurons, and if profound or prolonged it can cause irreversible brain damage. Repeated, though not necessarily prolonged, episodes of hypoglycemia may also be a source of hippocampal damage. I recently read a report about a ninety-six-year-old woman in Japan who suffered bouts of hypoglycemia after meals high in carbohydrate, and the authors of this paper remarked that this is common among the elderly of Japan. In some European hospitals, nearly 9 percent of elderly patients who do not have diabetes and are not receiving medications to artificially lower blood glucose suffer bouts of hypoglycemia. In many cases, this is due to poor liver function or adrenal exhaustion. However, in a significant number of cases this is due to poor tolerance of high-carbohydrate meals.

CARDIOVASCULAR DISEASE

Another major contributor to the risk of developing dementia is cardiovascular disease. There are three major ways in which cardiovascular disease manifests in the body. These include ischemic vascular disease, in which arteries in various tissues in the body become narrowed or blocked by fatty deposits; heart failure, in which the heart is no longer able to keep up with the body's demand for oxygen- and nutrient-carrying blood; and abnormal rhythms, when the normally regular, predictable beat of the heart becomes erratic. All three of these presentations of heart and artery disease have been found to increase the risk of dementia.

Ischemic vascular disease arises when the arteries that supply blood to the heart, brain, kidneys, and other organs begin to narrow. This narrowing is due to the accumulation of fatty material in the lining and inner layers of arteries in a disease process called atherosclerosis. Atherosclerosis begins when injuries to the lining of small arteries attract specialized cells to the damaged tissue. These cells, which include blood platelets and white blood cells, stick to the walls of damaged arteries. They secrete powerful substances to patch up leaks in the walls, protect the arteries from further damage, and start repair processes. The damage to the arteries need not be severe for the platelets and white blood cells to be called to the scene. High blood pressure, chemical insult from smoking, or even high levels of fat in the blood may be sufficient irritation to start the process. Unfortunately, these cells were intended to be called to defend the arteries in emergency situations, such as arteries being damaged by trauma or infections. They were not intended to be on constant duty. When they remain active on a persistent basis, the substances they release can begin to create conditions of chronic inflammation. It is this inflammation, in combination with high cholesterol and other unhealthy conditions in the blood, that start the process of atherosclerosis and scarring of the lining of the arteries in the brain and elsewhere in the body.

When the heart's own arteries, the coronary arteries, begin to narrow, discomfort called angina may be experienced during exertion. This pain arises when the needs of the heart muscle outpace its blood supply. As the condition progresses, plaques in the coronary arteries grow more likely to ulcerate and become sites of clot formation. The end result can be a heart attack, or what physicians call myocardial infarction. Several different procedures have been developed to restore blood flow to heart muscle that suffers from narrowed coronary arteries. The well-known coronary artery bypass grafting, or CABG procedure (pronounced "cabbage" by physicians), is one way to restore blood flow. Another is the insertion of a catheter up into the heart through the femoral artery in the groin. The catheter is then guided into the coronary arteries that branch off from the main artery in the body, the aorta. The coronary artery is then widened by being subjected to internal pressure by blowing up a small balloon that presses the fatty plaques flat against the walls of the artery. This procedure is called balloon angioplasty. There has been a long and bitter controversy in the medical literature about whether or not the CABG procedure, which often requires redirecting the patient's blood through a so-called heart-lung machine, is an independent source of brain damage, cognitive loss, and dementia in patients who undergo this procedure. The most recent reviews that I have read conclude that the risk of cognitive loss after CABG surgery is much less than had once been thought. Whether this is due to improvement in technique, more care in minimizing risk, or the use of less risky alternative methods such as balloon angioplasty in high-risk patients is not clear. If you have been told that you are a candidate for CABG surgery, then this is a topic to discuss with your physician.

Vascular dementia is the most obvious problem that can result from damage to arteries in the brain. This can occur after arteries that supply the brain are blocked or ruptured, which is what we refer to as having a stroke. This damage to cerebral blood vessels can also manifest in the form of Binswanger's disease, in which large areas of the subcortical brain are affected by diffuse damage to small arteries. The interference with blood supply in Binswanger's disease is usually a matter of chronic impairment, rather than complete loss as in stroke. The inflammation and reduced oxygen levels that occur within arteries due to atherosclerosis can also damage the brain indirectly, when chemical signals produced by these processes pass through the blood vessels and trigger chemical changes inside the brain that stimulate degenerative processes.

Heart failure is the inability of the heart to maintain output of blood sufficient to meet the body's changing needs. It can be due to loss of heart muscle following a heart attack, or to weakening of the heart after years of pumping blood against the resistance of high blood pressure. Heart failure has been associated with increased risk for dementia. Studies have shown that cognitive function decreases in parallel with decreases in heart function. This is due to the damaged heart's difficulty in pumping enough blood to the brain. People with heart failure also tend to have difficulty pumping blood through their lungs, which results in chronic states of inadequate oxygenation of the blood. This further deprives the brain of needed oxygen and triggers inflammatory processes in brain tissue. These effects are thought to exacerbate the neurodegenerative processes of dementia. When the heart begins to fail, the kidneys and liver begin to suffer as well. This leads to the buildup of toxins in the blood and the brain being deprived of the healthy environment it requires to function properly.

The muscle cells of the heart have the ability to beat on their own, with their own natural rhythm. The heart receives nerve impulses from the brain that can increase or decrease the heart rate, according to the body's needs. However, the heart also has its own, internal system of communication, a sort of nervous system, that allows its muscle cells to work together to beat in a smooth and controlled fashion. The heart's internal communication system can malfunction or break down. This can occur when tissue is damaged after a heart attack, in states of heart failure, or when hormonal or chemical abnormalities occur. When the normal regular beating of the heart is disrupted, several different adverse effects may result. An irregular, poorly coordinated heartbeat decreases the efficiency of the heart and creates problems that are essentially the same as those of heart failure. A smooth, regular beating motion also keeps blood moving properly through the heart. When normal rhythm is disrupted, blood can pool abnormally and begin to form clots. This exposes the person to risk of stroke if these clots break loose from the walls of heart, travel through the bloodstream, and lodge in the brain. A rather common form of faulty heart rhythm called atrial fibrillation is associated with increased risk of vascular dementia. Doctors treat patients with atrial fibrillation with medications that prevent clot formation and try, when possible, to restore normal rhythm. When the health of the heart begins to decline due to metabolic syndrome, stress, smoking, lack of exercise, and many other causes, the risk of dementia increases, and this can occur through a number of different mechanisms.

HOMOCYSTEINE, VITAMIN B$_{12}$, AND FOLIC ACID

Homocysteine is a natural substance in the body that is not harmful under normal circumstances. In fact, it is a necessary component of several important biochemical pathways in the body. However, homocysteine has recently come to be suspected of playing roles in the development of both cardiovascular disease and dementia. Studies have found that cognitive function varies inversely with blood levels of homocysteine. That is, when homocysteine levels go up, cognitive function can be expected to go down. However, this relationship is complicated, as hyperhomocysteinemia, the tongue-twisting technical term for high homocysteine, is both a symptom and a cause of problems. Homocysteine is made when the amino acid methionine gives up what is called a methyl group. The transfer of a methyl group from one molecule to another in the body is a common and extremely important reaction. Methionine performs this task in the form of S-adenosylmethionine, or SAMe, which I discuss in more detail in the chapter titled "Vitamins, Herbs, and Nutraceuticals." Some of the homocysteine that is produced in the methyl group transfer process is used to make other substances, such as the amino acid cysteine and the important antioxidant, glutathione. However, for the most part, the homocysteine is recycled back into methionine with the help of vitamin B$_{12}$ and folic acid. When vitamin B$_{12}$ and folic acid are deficient, homocysteine builds up. Thus, hyperhomocysteinemia is taken as a sign of a lack of one or both of these vitamins. A simple blood test can quickly determine whether or not an individual suffers from too much homocysteine.

Homocysteine may directly cause problems in the brain. In animals, the injection of homocysteine into the cerebrospinal fluid results in increases in hyperphosphorylation of tau protein, which in turn increases the formation of neurofibrillary tangles in Alzheimer's dementia. Moreover, whereas the Alzheimer's medication memantine blocks the activity of certain glutamate receptors in the brain, homocysteine appears to stimulate some of these receptors. The overstimulation of glutamate receptors in the brain can lead to over-excitation and cell death. There is also evidence that homocysteine can interfere with normal control of DNA involved in producing enzymes that process amyloid protein. A recent report even suggests that in laboratory rats, high levels of homocysteine may interfere with the process of neurogenesis, which produces new neurons and helps maintain cognitive function. Hyperhomocysteinemia is also a risk factor for cardiovascular disease, which in turn makes it a risk factor for vascular dementia. High levels of homocysteine are associated with small silent strokes and with white matter damage in the brain. To some extent, homocysteine may be a marker for other problems, such as vitamin deficiencies, that aggravate heart disease. However, there are many studies suggesting that homocysteine may itself adversely affect the function of the heart and arteries and thus directly increase the risk of heart disease, stroke, and dementia.

Deficiencies of vitamin B_{12} and/or folic acid have also long been seen as risk factors for dementia. Vitamin B_{12} is present in almost all foods of animal origin, such as meat, fish, eggs, and dairy products. Brewer's yeast or so-called nutritional yeast is another good source of this vitamin. Food of plant origin does not contain B_{12}. Unfortunately, it is possible to consume enough vitamin B_{12} in your diet yet still be deficient in the vitamin because of an inability to absorb it from the intestine. A substance from the stomach called "intrinsic factor" is needed to absorb B_{12}. If a person has stomach problems such as ulcers, gastritis, or certain stomach infections, the production of intrinsic factor may be impaired along with the ability to absorb vitamin B_{12}. People who have had gastric bypass surgery are often unable to absorb B_{12}, and they must receive shots or high doses of it in pill form. I have found an astonishing number of elderly people to have low vitamin B_{12} levels, despite the fact that they have a primary care doctor and receive regular medical checkups.

Folic acid is found in almost all plant sources of food, as well as in eggs, liver, and other organ meats. Despite its availability, deficiencies in folic acid are quite common. Individuals who take certain medications, particularly ones to prevent seizures, need extra amounts of folate to prevent deficiency. Thankfully, it is very easy to determine the blood levels of both B_{12} and folic acid. Because these deficiencies are common and contribute to dementia as well as major depression and other psychiatric illnesses, I quite often send my patients to the laboratory to have their levels of these vitamins measured.

One of the ways that deficiencies of these vitamins can cause dementia is by increasing blood levels of homocysteine. However, when you lack these vitamins, you also lack the ability to regenerate methionine out of that homocysteine. A lack of methionine deprives the body of one of the major sources of methyl groups needed by the brain and other tissues of the body. In the brain, the S-adenosylmethionine form of methionine supplies methyl groups to make neurotransmitters, including acetylcholine. Transfer of methyl groups also plays a role in turning on and off DNA that controls processes such as amyloid protein metabolism and programmed cell death, or apoptosis.

Another function of vitamin B_{12} is to produce substances used in making DNA. Therefore, its deficiency most clearly affects cells that divide and grow rapidly, such as blood cells. It is not known if B_{12} deficiency affects neurogenesis in the brain, but I would not be surprised if it did. It is known that some rapidly growing cells in the brain that wrap around neuron bundles and insulate the electrical impulses in them can be affected by B_{12} deficiency. Breakdown of this insulating material can cause dementia-like signs and symptoms. Vitamin B_{12} is also involved in bringing the metabolic products of the breakdown of certain amino acids into the mitochondria to be burned in a chemical reaction known as the Krebs cycle. One of these breakdown products, methylmalonic acid, is toxic to the brain. Vitamin B_{12} deficiency causes an increase in this toxic substance, which then causes damage to the brain.

Although vitamin B_{12} deficiency can cause cognitive disturbance, if it is diagnosed early enough, it can be treated and reversed. This is quite different from Alzheimer's and other neurodegenerative forms of dementia. Deficiency of vitamin B_{12} is not as closely associated with Alzheimer's dementia, per se, as is deficiency of folic acid. Folic acid deficiency has been found to disrupt enzymes that process amyloid, and thus to increase beta amyloid deposition in the brains of normal mice. In another study, low folate, but not low B_{12}, correlated with high levels of hyperphosphorylated tau protein in cerebrospinal fluid. This may further suggest that low folate may participate in producing an Alzheimer's-like dementia.

"LAST ONE IN IS A ROTTEN EGG!"

One of the most fascinating and fruitful discoveries in the past ten years has been the finding that some simple gases, including several extremely toxic ones, serve critical chemical messenger functions in the human brain. Scientists were surprised when nitric oxide was found to serve as a neurotransmitter in the brain. They were astonished when the poisonous gas carbon monoxide (CO) was characterized as a natural and important chemical modulator of brain activity. The gas most recently added to this list of unlikely chemical messengers is hydrogen sulfide (H_2S). H_2S provides much of the charming fragrance of rotten eggs. Gram for gram, H_2S is more deadly than CO. If breathed in concentrations as dilute as 500 parts per million, H_2S can bring a miserable and malodorous death. However, when a substance is poisonous, it is often because it plugs into an existing chemical system of communication in the body. This appears to be the case with H_2S.

It has long been known that H_2S exists in relatively high concentration in brain and other tissues in the body. When the reason for such levels of this noxious gas was explored, it was discovered that the brain actually produces its own H_2S molecules. The brain possesses all of the chemical machinery it needs to perform this task. The enzyme cystathionine beta-synthase (CBS), with the help of pyridoxine (vitamin B_6), converts the amino acid cysteine into H_2S. This reaction is facilitated by interaction with S-adenosylmethionine, which I discuss to some extent above and will explore in more detail later.

H_2S is now known to have several important effects in the brain. It enhances activity at the NMDA receptor that takes part in the process called "long term potentiation," or LTP. LTP is necessary for learning and memory. H_2S has important antioxidant and anti-inflammatory effects in brain tissue. H_2S also acts in the hypothalamus of the brain to dampen release of a hormone called corticotropin-releasing hormone (CRH). CRH is one of the triggers that leads to stimulation of the adrenal glands to release the stress hormone cortisol. Thus, deficiency of H_2S synthesis can exacerbate the stress response. The CBS enzyme is also involved in one of the pathways that rids brain tissue of homocysteine. Thus, underactivity of the enzyme can increase concentrations of homocysteine in the brain and other tissues of the body. Adequate CBS activity is important enough for the health of the brain that certain genetic abnormalities in the structure of the enzyme have now been recognized as risk factors for the development of Alzheimer's dementia.

H_2S levels have been found to be abnormally low in the brains of people diagnosed with Alzheimer's dementia. Conversely, studies in animals have found that enhancing H_2S synthesis decreases the damage caused by beta amyloid in brain cells. H_2S protects brain cells from the oxidative stress and inflammation that amyloid generates, and it helps mitochondria maintain their function in cells threatened by amyloid deposition.

It is possible that deficient levels of B_{12}, folate, and S-adenosylmethionine may further contribute to dementia by impairing the flow of sulfur-containing amino acids into the synthesis of H_2S. A lack of vitamin B_6 would even further impair this process. On the other hand, sulfur-containing substances in plants, particularly garlic and onions, may reduce the risk of dementia, in part by increasing the raw materials to produce more H_2S in the brain and bloodstream.

MITOCHONDRIAL FAILURE

Mitochondria are the powerhouses of cells, including neurons in the brain. They produce the energy-storing molecules of adenosine triphosphate (ATP) that drive all cellular activity. Animal cells, including those of humans, are utterly dependent on the energy produced by the mitochondria, and when the mitochondria cease to function, the cell dies.

A fascinating theory in modern biology is that the mitochondria in our cells were at one time separate, bacteria-like creatures. Early in the evolution of life they invaded and later became symbiotic components of larger cellular life forms. In some respects, mitochondria are alien life forms that took up residence in our ancestors and were passed down to us. This theory is known as the endosymbiotic hypothesis. One of the strongest arguments for the endosymbiotic hypothesis is that mitochondria have their own, unique form of DNA that is separate from the DNA in the nucleus of the cells they inhabit. In fact, unlike the coiled strands of DNA in the nucleus of our cells, mitochondrial DNA is circular, like that found in many primitive bacteria.

Sperm cells from our fathers carry mitochondria in their tails. However the tails of sperm cells break off before the sperm and egg merge to initiate embryo development; thus all of the mitochondria in our bodies come from our mother's egg cell. Mitochondria, as well as a growing list of mitochondrial diseases, are passed on entirely by the mother. Through the hundreds of millions of years that mitochondria have made their home in cells, they have become literally a part of the cell. In fact, while they have their own unique form of DNA, roughly 90 percent of the proteins in mitochondria are coded for by DNA in the nucleus of the cell and not by their own DNA. Because the mitochondria are entirely dependent on the cell for nurturance, the major portion of their protein, and raw materials for their activities, mitochondria can in fact suffer from cellular problems inherited from the father. Still, by and large, if your mother's mitochondria are strong and resilient, yours are too.

Paradoxically, the chemical activities that are carried out in the mitochondria are not only critical for life, but also a continuous threat to it.

A complex assembly line of molecules has the responsibility of passing extremely reactive electrons down the electron transport chain to finally generate the all-important ATP. Along the way, a number of very reactive and toxic compounds are unavoidably produced. These dangerous substances are referred to as reactive oxygen species (ROS). Cells in the body have ways of neutralizing the dangers of ROS, including enzymes that convert ROS to less destructive molecules and antioxidants that buffer cells and their component parts from oxidative stress. Some antioxidants, such as alpha-lipoic acid, are made in the body, whereas others, such as vitamins E and C, must be consumed as part of the diet. Protection of mitochondria is one way in which antioxidants help maintain the health of cells in the body, including neurons in the brain.

In metabolic syndrome, the body begins to lose control of the burning and proper storage of fat. Fat can also begin to collect inside the mitochondria. Not only does this accumulation of fat interfere with the finely tuned biochemical processes that take place in the mitochondria, but it carries the same risks as placing your wood pile right next to the fireplace in your living room. Fat is dangerous material, and it is very easily oxidized. This abnormal process, called lipid peroxidation, is yet another source of ROS and destructive processes inside the mitochondria that lead to loss of mitochondrial function and cell death.

Amyloid protein, as is produced in excess in Alzheimer's dementia, may also collect inside mitochondria. This deposition of amyloid in the mitochondria initiates a vicious cycle in neurons in the brain. The amyloid disrupts the mitochondria's ability to contain the dangerous electron transport reactions that unleash ROS. The ROS diffuse into the cell, flipping the "on" switches for genetic machinery in the nuclei of neurons that, along with triggering a variety of other inflammatory and defensive processes, leads to the production of even more aberrant amyloid protein.

Abnormalities in mitochondrial function, some of which may be inherited through maternal mitochondrial DNA, have been implicated in mental illnesses including major depression, bipolar affective disorder, and schizophrenia. There have also been suggestions in the scientific literature that certain types of inherited mitochondrial DNA may predispose people to Alzheimer's and other forms of dementia. However, there has yet to be a strong connection made between any specific type of mitochondrial DNA and dementia. It is possible that certain forms of mitochondrial DNA make dementia more likely only if inflammation, oxidative stress, or other factors are also present. In any case, it is clear that mitochondrial dysfunction does play a role in the development of dementia, and that inflammation, high blood glucose levels, oxidative stress, and other factors seen in metabolic syndrome are largely responsible for the initial mitochondrial damage. Fortunately, along with taking steps to avoid metabolic syndrome, there are ways to protect mitochondria from these damaging effects, as well as ways to enhance their activity to help prevent dementia. In the chapter on supplementation with herbs, vitamins, and nutraceuticals, I discuss a number of substances that can be used for this purpose.

MAJOR DEPRESSION

A history of major depression increases the risk of developing dementia. The risk of Alzheimer's dementia is roughly doubled in people with long histories of depression in their adult lives. In fact, depression in middle age has been found to continue to increase the risk of dementia as much as twenty-five years later. Patients with Alzheimer's who also suffer major depression have more amyloid plaques and neurofibrillary tangles in their brains than do Alzheimer's patients without depression. If people are diagnosed as having MCI, their likelihood of progressing to true dementia is roughly doubled if they also have major depression. Suffering depression at the time a patient is first diagnosed with Alzheimer's dementia is associated with needing placement in a nursing home or other care facility sooner than if the patient had not been suffering depression.

It is not uncommon for people in the early stages of dementia to become depressed. In some cases, this is due to a subtle awareness that their minds are slipping away. However, the chronic state of not being able to do all of the things one used to do and enjoy can itself bring a sense of boredom and despondency. In some cases, patients in the early stages of Alzheimer's dementia begin to feel depressed without any obvious reasons why. This may reflect the fact that some of the abnormal changes that occur in brain tissue in the neurodegenerative processes of dementia may themselves generate symptoms of major depression. Depression can be the first visible tip of the dementia iceberg, with many patients reporting significant changes in their mood in the year or two prior to the diagnosis of their dementia.

Although major depression and Alzheimer's dementia often overlap, it has been difficult to discern if major depression causes Alzheimer's dementia, or if changes occurring in the brains of patients with Alzheimer's bring on the symptoms of depression. In all likelihood, both these possibilities are true. Nonetheless, there is scientific evidence that having episodes of major depression in younger adult life can increase the risks of developing

Alzheimer's and vascular dementia many years later. What is it about major depression that increases the risk of dementia?

A common view of major depression is that it is merely a set of feelings and thoughts that grow out of loss and disappointment. Certainly, an episode of major depression can arise in an otherwise cheerful person after he or she unexpectedly suffers great personal loss. The death of a loved one, serious illness, divorce, losing a job, or having a home and belongings destroyed in a natural disaster are all events that can be expected to precipitate an episode of major depression in many people who had previously never experienced this illness. Unfortunately, the so-called golden years are years in which many great personal losses tend to occur. I have seen many strong men fall into a downward spiral when they retire. Their jobs were more important to their sense of self-esteem than they had ever realized. They can feel useless and bored. Being at work may also have provided a bit of a buffer zone between husband and wife, and marital problems can erupt when more time is spent together. A person's sixties and seventies can be years in which illnesses that have long been smoldering flame up in full intensity. Financial problems can arise when fixed incomes cannot be stretched to meet the demands of new health problems, expensive medications, and doctor visits. This is also a time when ill health can take the life of a spouse, with women more often than men being left to carry on.

Despite the many losses and stresses that can befall people as they enter the later stages of their lives, I often see patients who tell me that they can't understand why they feel so depressed when everything in their life is so great. This points to the fact that in many cases, major depression begins as a problem in brain chemistry. The biological nature of major depression is revealed by the evidence that some people are genetically predisposed to depression. This is most evident in studies of depression in identical and fraternal twins. When one of a pair of identical twins suffers major depression, it is nearly twice as likely that the other twin will also suffer depression than is the case with fraternal twins. It is important to note, however, that the concordance rate for diagnosis of depression among sets of identical twins is not 100 percent. Thus, genes do not guarantee that a person will either suffer or be free from major depression. All in all, studies have shown that genes contribute about 40 percent of the risk for developing major depression.

An underappreciated fact about major depression is that the entire body is affected. Many people with depression have chemical markers of inflammation and high levels of cortisol in their blood. High blood levels of cortisol are associated with increased risk for developing Alzheimer's dementia.

Sleep cycles and appetite are also disturbed in major depression, and the resulting loss of sleep and deficits in nutrition can further increase the risk of dementia.

Most antidepressants cause an increase in brain levels of brain-derived neurotrophic factor, or BDNF, and in the rate of production of new neurons through the process of neurogenesis. Thus, it has been suspected that decreases in levels of BDNF and the rate of neurogenesis may be a hallmark of major depression as well as playing an important role in causing dementia. In fact, the hippocampus is an area that is both exquisitely sensitive to the stimulatory effects of BDNF and the location of most neurogenesis in the brain. The hippocampus shrinks in the brains of individuals who have a long history of depression, and this shrinkage in size is in direct correlation with the length of the depressive illness. The hippocampus is also one of the earliest victims of degenerative change in Alzheimer's dementia. It is no coincidence that high levels of cortisol and inflammation, low BDNF, and decreased rates of neurogenesis, which all exacerbate major depression, also appear to play a role in the development of Alzheimer's and other forms of dementia.

Major depression further increases the risk of dementia by increasing the likelihood of cardiovascular disease. Major depression independently contributes to all three major forms of heart disease, including heart failure, abnormal heart rhythms, and atherosclerosis. Adults with depression are two to three times as likely to later be diagnosed with heart disease than are people without depression. It has recently been shown that simply having a pessimistic outlook on life increases the risk of death from heart disease.

Over recent years it has also become apparent that there are relationships between major depression, metabolic syndrome, and diabetes. Metabolic syndrome can increase the risk for major depression; however, statistical studies have shown that the more usual progression is from depression to metabolic syndrome, and then often to heart disease and diabetes. Overeating, smoking, drinking, inactivity, and carbohydrate craving are at least partially responsible for the tendency of people with depression to develop metabolic syndrome. However, even when these unhealthy habits are statistically removed from the equation, there is an unexpectedly high incidence of metabolic syndrome among sufferers of major depression. It is likely that the inflammatory processes, abdominal obesity, and increased levels of cortisol in major depression contribute to the progression of metabolic syndrome.

There is also a strong relationship between depression and insulin resistance. Insulin resistance, the cardinal feature of metabolic syndrome, is four times more likely to occur in depressed individuals. When insulin resistance is found in the body, it is likely to exist in brain tissue as well. Insulin resistance in brain tissue may exacerbate both major depression and various forms of dementia.

It is important to treat major depression early after its presentation. After all, life is short, and being depressed is a tragic way to spend one's brief time here on Earth. If it is possible to prevent or delay dementia by treating depression, then so much the better. Unfortunately, once a patient with depression is diagnosed as also having Alzheimer's dementia, studies show treatment of the depression by standard methods does little to alter the course of the dementia.

OBESITY

There is growing evidence that being obese increases one's risk for developing dementia. In one study, abdominal obesity in middle-aged subjects predicted an increased risk of developing Alzheimer's dementia more than thirty years later. Unfortunately, obesity is yet another health problem that is growing to epidemic proportions. It is estimated that up to 40 percent of adults in the United States are obese, with the prevalence rate growing. Of particular concern is the growing prevalence of obesity among children and adolescents. It is likely that we are setting the stage for an explosion in future rates of heart disease, diabetes, and dementia.

To some degree, the risk of dementia goes up with obesity because sufferers are so likely to have other well-known risk factors for dementia, such as metabolic syndrome, diabetes, cardiovascular disease, sleep apnea, and inflammatory processes. The coexistence of obesity with all of these other factors is consistent with the fact that abdominal obesity, the pot-bellied extra storage of fat around the abdominal organs, is the type of obesity associated with both Alzheimer's dementia and metabolic syndrome. Nonetheless, there are studies suggesting that obesity in midlife may predispose a person to dementia apart from diabetes and cardiovascular disease. Even in young men and women in their forties who are obese but otherwise healthy, abnormalities can be seen in the white matter in many areas of the brain. These abnormal changes are particularly marked in the frontal lobes, and they are thought to represent accelerated aging of the brain. It is not clear why this happens. It is possible that some of the adipocytokines released from visceral fat cells have adverse effects on the brain even before they produce such effects on the heart and metabolic function.

I should note that being significantly underweight also appears to be a risk factor developing dementia. This may be due to co-morbid illnesses or overall ill health of people who are severely underweight.

SLEEP APNEA AND INADEQUATE SLEEP

The risk of Alzheimer's and vascular dementias is increased in people who have a history of sleep apnea. In fact, as many as 70 percent of patients with Alzheimer's disease also have sleep apnea. Sleep apnea is a cessation of breathing during sleep. To be diagnosed as sleep apnea, these episodes of not breathing must last for ten seconds or more. About 5 percent of adults in the United States are diagnosed with sleep apnea. However, sleep apnea is woefully underdiagnosed, and as many as 31 percent of men and 21 percent of women meet criteria that place them at high risk for this condition.

In obstructive apnea, the most common form of sleep apnea, the airway collapses during sleep and breathing is mechanically stopped. The most obvious reason the airway is blocked is that muscles of the throat lose tone during sleep and no longer keep fatty tissue from bulging into the air passage. Obesity is well known to increase the risk of obstructive sleep apnea. However, not everyone with sleep apnea is obese. Another cause of sleep apnea is loss of tone of the muscles of the tongue during sleep. Even in people without obesity, this can result in the tongue falling back into the throat and blocking the airway. This is particularly likely to occur if a person sleeps on his or her back. In fact, for some individuals, simply switching to sleeping on their sides can eliminate or greatly reduce the problem.

Sleep apnea is complex in that it causes two separate problems. One is a drop in blood oxygen levels, which is called hypoxia, and the other is loss of sleep. The hypoxia caused by cessation of breathing damages fine capillaries that supply the brain with blood. This damage paves the way for the subcortical ischemic type of vascular dementia, such as Binswanger's dementia, and increases the ability of blood to clot in arteries, which increases the risk of stroke. The lack of oxygen also precipitates degenerative processes that are similar to those seen in Alzheimer's and other dementias. Hypoxia is known to stimulate the enzyme GSK-3 in the brain. This is the enzyme that is inhibited by insulin and that tends to be overactive in metabolic syndrome. GSK-3 stimulates inflammation, hyperphosphorylation of tau, neurofibrillary tangles, amyloid deposition, and helps trigger apoptosis, the program of cellular suicide. Studies in mice have shown that hypoxia stimulates the production of the abnormal amyloid protein that accumulates in the brain tissues of patients with Alzheimer's. Ironically, hypoxia also increases the production of destructive reactive oxygen species. This is likely due to the fact that oxygen-deprived cells are no longer able to manage safe burning of fuel in the mitochondria, nor are they able to mount a strong defense to safely rid themselves of the reactive oxygen species that are an inevitable byproduct of metabolism. These reactive molecules further stimulate inflammation and cell death, which contribute to dementia.

Hypoxia is a severe stress that increases serum levels of the stress hormone cortisol. Persistently high levels of cortisol can cause damage to neurons in the brain, and this damage is likely additive to that of the pathological processes at work in Alzheimer's and other dementias. Cortisol also plays a role in regulating the sleep cycle. Thus, the hypercortisolemia of sleep apnea may further contribute to sleep disturbance.[5]

In sleep apnea, blood oxygen levels fall intermittently throughout the night. In response to these low oxygen levels, the brain struggles to awaken and stimulate breathing. During such an episode, a sufferer may partially awaken for a few seconds and quickly fall back into sleep without being aware of it. In severe cases, this can occur hundreds of times throughout the night. Consequently, it is not uncommon for individuals with sleep apnea to report sleeping through the night but waking up in the morning more exhausted than when they went to bed.

When deprived of sleep we feel tired. We have difficulty concentrating and performing our usual daily activities. However, along with the subjective experience of fatigue and mental strain, the body reacts to sleep deprivation as it would to any other disruption of normal function. Simply restricting the amount of sleep one gets, even without the hypoxia of sleep apnea, stimulates release of cortisol. Too little sleep also activates the sympathetic nervous system, which mediates the "fight or flight" response. Sympathetic nervous system activation raises blood pressure and, particularly in the presence of high levels of cortisol, causes increases in blood glucose levels. Chemical markers of inflammation also begin to rise in the blood after a person has been deprived of a full night's sleep for a prolonged period of

---

5. Ordinarily, the lowest cortisol levels of the day occur at about midnight, whereas the highest levels of the hormone occur around six to eight o'clock in the morning. It is thought that these relatively high levels of cortisol in the morning help a person wake up, as well as feel hungry for breakfast. People who suffer major depression often exhibit poor regulation of their serum cortisol, and tend to have hypercortisolemia, or high cortisol levels. The well-known phenomenon of what psychiatrists call early morning awakening in people suffering major depression is most likely due to early and increased release of cortisol.

time. Obesity is yet another problem that can result from a chronic lack of adequate sleep. This may be due to the fact that inadequate sleep alters levels of several important hormones, including leptin and ghrelin, that help control appetite.

So far, there is no concrete evidence that inadequate sleep increases the risk of dementia. However, inadequate sleep has been shown to increase the risk of metabolic syndrome, diabetes type 2, hypercortisolemia, obesity, and major depression, each of which does increase the risk of developing dementia. A recent study published in the *Journal of the American Medical Association* showed a strong relationship between inadequate sleep and the risk of developing coronary artery disease. The coronary arteries are the vessels by which the heart provides its own blood supply, and blockage of these arteries is the cause of heart attacks. Calcium deposits in the walls of coronary arteries, which could later lead to heart attacks, were three times more likely to occur in people who slept fewer than five hours a night than in those who slept six or more hours. What is particularly alarming about this data is that the subjects who participated were all healthy, young adults in their thirties and forties. None of them had been found to have evidence of calcification of their coronary arteries prior to the start of the five-year study. Coronary artery disease can, albeit indirectly, increase the risk of dementia. It was not determined if inadequate sleep led to calcification of the walls of small arteries serving the brain similar to what was seen in coronary arteries. However, if this is the case, then inadequate sleep would almost certainly increase the risk of vascular dementia in a far more direct fashion.

Unfortunately, over the past forty years, the average American has been getting one and half to two hours less sleep a night than they used to. The number of young adults getting less than seven hours of sleep a night has doubled within that time. Altered sleep patterns, such as working at night rather than during the usual 9 a.m. to 5 p.m. period, may produce some of the same effects as loss of sleep. The epidemic of inadequate sleep may thus be contributing to the epidemic of dementia.

STRESS AND CORTISOL

Most people use the word stress to mean the physical strain and emotional pressure we feel when dealing with difficult problems in our lives. However, doctors see stress as a more complicated phenomenon. When we are pushed beyond our usual capacities, the brain initiates a series of chemical signals that prepares the body to deal with the extra demands we are facing. Earlier in evolution, this extra demand might have been escaping from a saber-toothed tiger or fighting to win a mate. In modern society, it is more likely to be an IRS audit or a nasty divorce proceeding. Nonetheless, the body's response to stress remains the same as it always has.

A major component of this response is the release of the hormone cortisol from the adrenal glands. Cortisol is a glucocorticoid. This term is derived from the fact that one of the primary functions of cortisol is to maintain adequate serum glucose levels during the fasting state and to help provide a boost of energy under stressful situations. It enhances serum glucose levels by stimulating the breakdown of protein and facilitating the transformation of the resulting amino acids into glucose in the liver. Cortisol also acts in the brain to increase the production of necessary neurotransmitters to allow the brain to function under trying circumstances.

Cortisol is essential for adequate responses to the normal stresses of life. However, high concentrations of cortisol are meant for emergencies, and not for day-to-day maintenance of the body. When cortisol is elevated for prolonged periods of time, the body and brain begin to suffer damage. Among the problems that can occur due to prolonged periods of stress are obesity, impairment of the immune system, atherosclerosis, and osteoporosis. Prolonged high levels of cortisol can also cause depression, likely due to changes it can cause in brain chemistry and structure.

There is also compelling evidence that exposure to high concentrations of cortisol for long periods of time contributes to Alzheimer's dementia and can make the disease progress more rapidly. People with Alzheimer's dementia tend to have high levels of cortisol in their blood. They also have high levels of cortisol in their cerebrospinal fluid. Of course, Alzheimer's, and every other form of dementia, can be an extremely distressing condition for the person suffering the illness. Thus, it is reasonable to wonder if the increase in cortisol that is generally seen in the blood of demented patients helps cause the illness, or if it is simply the result of the stress patients experience as the illness progresses. Although both scenarios are likely to occur, there are studies that suggest that in many cases high cortisol may come first. In one such study, cortisol levels of high-functioning adults between seventy and seventy-nine years of age were measured, and their cognitive performance was measured three and seven years later. The group of initially normal individuals with the highest levels of cortisol were the ones most likely to show cognitive decline over the following seven years. In another study, cognitive function of normal, elderly adults was measured along with psychological studies to determine their lifelong tendency to develop distress when under pressure. Those with the greatest tendency to develop distress, which in turn would have likely increased blood cortisol levels, were also more likely to develop Alzheimer's dementia.

The only sure way to determine if high levels of cortisol cause Alzheimer's would be to administer high doses of cortisol to some high-functioning adults, but not to others, and see if more cases of Alzheimer's dementia develop in the group that received the cortisol. Such an unethical experiment could never be performed with human subjects. However, such studies have been performed using laboratory animals. Administration of high concentrations of the rodent equivalent of cortisol, corticosterone, increases deposits of abnormal forms of amyloid and tau protein, just as is seen in the brains of patients with Alzheimer's dementia. Chronic stress, which stimulates the adrenal glands to release corticosterone into the blood, also causes increases of amyloid deposition in the brains of mice genetically engineered to produce the human form of amyloid precursor protein.

High levels of cortisol may also independently cause deficits in cognitive function that could make dementia worse. Neurons are structurally complicated cells. One of their characteristics is sending out projections that resemble the branches of trees. The finest of these branches, which are called dendrites, come into close contact with other neurons and serve as a means to receive chemical messages from those neighboring cells. Activity in neurons tends to increase the complexity of the dendritic branching, and, in turn, a lot of dendritic branching facilitates complex activity such as learning and cognitive processing. High levels of cortisol, generated either by direct administration of large doses or by subjection of animals to high degrees of stress, has been found to prune back dendritic branching and, ostensibly, to reduce the ability of neurons to process complex information. It is known for example, that cortisol decreases the ability of neurons in the hippocampus to lay down new memories. This may be the reason that people with conditions associated with high levels of cortisol, including not only Alzheimer's dementia, but also major depression and Cushing's disease, a condition where the adrenal glands pump out too much cortisol, have significant deficits in memory.

Cortisol may also diminish cognitive function by slowing or stopping neurogenesis. For years it was believed that when neurons in the brain die, they are gone and not replaced. However, in recent years it has been discovered that new neurons are constantly being born to replenish the supply of healthy neurons. This process of replenishing neurons is called neurogenesis. Neurogenesis occurs in the brains of all mammals, including humans. Both severe stress and administration of high doses of cortisol or corticosterone impairs neurogenesis. Chronic exposure to high levels of cortisol also makes neurons more vulnerable to the toxic effects of amyloid and other insults to the brain. Thus, cortisol both increases the likelihood of neuronal death and decreases the likelihood that the neuron will be replaced.

Exposure to cortisol causes certain areas of the brain, including the hippocampus, to shrink. This is seen in experimental animals given corticosterone or subjected to high stress. This shrinkage of the hippocampus is also seen in people with severe and persistent depression, post-traumatic stress disorder (PTSD), and Alzheimer's dementia. The shrinkage is likely due to both dying back of dendrites and the loss of neurogenesis to replenish cells that have died. The only bright side to the cortisol story is that many of the adverse effects of cortisol on the brain can be reversed if levels of the hormone are returned to normal. Of course, it is likely that a point of no return can be reached when damage is no longer reversible.

ESTROGEN

Whereas roughly 20 percent of men will develop dementia during their lifetime, it will occur in nearly 33 percent of women. In fact, simply being female has been considered to be a risk factor for developing dementia. It has long been suspected that decreases in estrogen that occur with menopause may be at least partially responsible for the higher rate of Alzheimer's dementia in women. However, the role of estrogen in protecting the brain from dementia remains puzzling and controversial.

The term "estrogen" does not refer to a specific hormone, but rather a family of related ovarian hormones that generate estrus, which is the time of fertility that occurs in female animals. The three main estrogen hormones in the human body are estradiol, estriol, and estrone. In young women who are still having there menstrual cycles, there is usually more estradiol than estrone. In postmenopausal women, levels of all of the estrogens are substantially decreased in the blood, with the highest levels remaining being those of estrone. The estrone in postmenopausal women is released from the adrenal glands rather than the ovaries. The third major estrogen, estriol, is highest in the blood of women who are pregnant. Interestingly, most of the estriol in pregnancy is produced not by the woman herself, but by the placenta, which is derived from fetal tissue. Estriol is not as potent as estradiol or estrone. In fact, estriol may even have some effects opposite of the other estrogens.

As is often the case in biology, the estrogen hormones have evolved to serve many roles in the body, including some that have little to do with fertility and sexual behaviors. Estrogens have a number of effects that would be expected to help protect the brain from Alzheimer's dementia. Estrogens decrease production of amyloid protein, prevent the hyperphosphorylation of tau protein that leads to neurofibrillary tangles, maintain growth of neurons, and protect against oxidative damage.

There is some "naturalistic" evidence that estrogens offer women protection from dementia, particularly dementia of the Alzheimer's type. Women who reach menopause late in life tend to exhibit less cognitive decline as they age. Although menopause causes a profound drop in the blood levels of estradiol and estrone, measurable amounts of these hormones continue to circulate in the blood in postmenopausal women, even when they are not receiving hormone replacement therapy. Postmenopausal women with higher levels of estradiol and estrone in their blood are better able to maintain cognitive function and are at lower risk of developing MCI or dementia.

There is also some puzzling, and somewhat contradictory, data suggesting that the likelihood of a woman developing Alzheimer's dementia may be affected by the number of times she has been pregnant. Several studies have shown that women who have never been pregnant are at lower risk for developing Alzheimer's dementia. During pregnancy, the relatively weak estrogen, estriol, is predominant, and some of the effects of this hormone are even counteracted by high levels of another female hormone, progesterone. Furthermore, for a year or so after delivery, women's estrogen levels tend to stay low, and women who have had children tend to continue to have relatively low levels of estrogen throughout their remaining reproductive years. The apparent protective effect of nulliparity, the technical term for not having had children, has been attributed to persistently higher levels of estrogens throughout such a woman's life prior to menopause. There are also epidemiological studies showing that women who have been diagnosed with Alzheimer's dementia tended to have been pregnant more times than those women without the diagnosis.

However, there are discrepancies in the literature. For example, a study from Finland found that women who were "grand parous," a quaint term for having had more than five full-term pregnancies, were somewhat *less* likely to develop Alzheimer's than woman who had carried fewer than five pregnancies to term. Women who were "grand grand parous," that is, who had carried more than ten pregnancies to term, were even less likely to go on to suffer Alzheimer's dementia. These rather confusing pieces of data may be explained by the presence of the APOE4 gene, stress, or education and other social factors. It has further been suspected that women who bear children late in life may be at increased risk for Alzheimer's dementia. However, several studies have found this not to be the case.

The Women's Health Initiative was a large study started in 1996 that was intended to discover what if any health benefits could be gained by women being given replacement hormones when their own natural estrogen declined at menopause. One among many questions pursued was whether or not estrogen replacement could decrease the risk of Alzheimer's dementia in postmenopausal women. Because estrogen without the added effects of progesterone can greatly increase the risk of uterine cancer, women in this study were treated with an estrogenic preparation called conjugated equine estrogen along with a progesterone-like synthetic hormone called medroxyprogesterone acetate. The family of estrogens found in conjugated equine estrogens is the dihydroequilins. The equestrians among you may recognize that *equine* refers to the fact that this is the type of estrogen found in horses. In all fairness, while the use of horse estrogen to treat women sounds extraordinarily unnatural, studies show that the dihydroequine estrogens act in a manner very similar to estradiol in the human female. Nonetheless, much to the shock of researchers, initial results from the overall study showed that women on hormone replacement with dihydroequilins were showing increased likelihood of coronary events, stroke, breast cancer, and pulmonary embolism. The study was stopped in 2002.

Although the hormone treatments were suspended, there was enough data collected from the six years of the Women's Health Initiative to draw conclusions about the effects of estrogen and progesterone on the risk of developing dementia in these women. Again, researchers were shocked. Women who received conjugated equine estrogen and medroxyprogesterone treatment had nearly twice the rate of developing Alzheimer's dementia as did women who simply received placebos. This startling finding led to the conclusion that estrogen and progesterone together increase the risk of Alzheimer's dementia.

Many physicians cringe at the phrase "bioidentical hormones." Nonetheless, while the phrase is awkward and appeals to a sense of magic and drama, it is the fault of medical and pharmaceutical communities that such distinctions need to be made. The term bioidentical simply refers to replacement of the lost natural hormones with the same, identical substances rather than synthetic molecules or merely similar versions from other species. It is not unreasonable to suspect that the dihydroequilins given to women for hormone replacement therapy do not fully replace the benefits of natural human estrogens. Moreover, it is possible that they add adverse effects that the natural hormones do not produce.

All in all, the jury is still out concerning what if any benefit women might receive from a carefully applied form of estrogen replacement therapy at menopause. It is possible that "bioidentical" estrogen and progesterone may be more effective and less injurious than equine estrogens and medroxyprogesterone preparations. Another important consideration is the fact that the degenerative processes of Alzheimer's dementia begin many years before they become apparent in a person's behavior. Thus, any period of time between menopause and start of replacement therapy that women go without sufficient estrogen may initiate or exacerbate degenerative processes that manifest years later and can't be overcome by starting hormone replacement years after menopause begins. Maintenance of levels of *natural* hormones without a menopausal lapse in levels may provide women some protection from Alzheimer's dementia. This is a very active and important area of research.

TESTOSTERONE

Although less dramatic than the decline of estrogen levels seen in women when they reach menopause, men also experience decreases in levels of testosterone as they age. As with estrogen, testosterone has neuroprotective effects in the brain, including an ability to reduce the abnormal production of amyloid and the hyperphosphorylation of tau protein. There is also evidence that testosterone may offer some protection against Alzheimer's and other forms of dementia. Low levels of testosterone are associated with increased risk for Alzheimer's dementia, as well as more benign age-related memory loss. Testosterone replacement therapy in men with low levels of testosterone improves memory and visuospatial performance. However, in men already diagnosed with Alzheimer's dementia, testosterone replacement improved quality of life but did not significantly improve cognitive function. Perhaps the damage was already done.

The complexity of how testosterone acts in the body is seen in the fact that while low levels of hormone may be harmful in most men, in those with the APOE4 protein, lower levels of testosterone may actually reduce some risk of Alzheimer's dementia. Any thoughts of treating men with testosterone must also be tempered by the fact that it is not yet clear whether it is testosterone or a derivative of the hormone that increases risk for prostate cancer. In any case, the seriousness of adverse effects of testosterone-like hormones should also give pause to anyone considering augmenting testosterone levels in the hope of improving cognitive function. Competent medical supervision is essential.

INFLAMMATION

Inflammation is a major contributor to the initiation and progression of all of the major forms of dementia. A recent study in the *Journal of the American Medical Association* showed that while Metabolic Syndrome increases the risk of dementia, this is particularly the case in people who also show signs of suffering inflammatory processes. Inflammation is a series of chemical and cellular reactions the body performs in its attempt to defend itself against a variety of insults. The Roman physician Celsus described the signs of inflammation in the first century, and his observations are still taught in medical schools today. The four classic signs of inflammation are *calor* (heat), *rubor* (redness), *tumor* (swelling), and *dolor* (pain). The red skin of sunburn, the swelling and pain of a bee sting, and the blotchy, itchy skin of hives are all examples of simple inflammatory responses.

Many inflammatory responses in irritated tissues involve the release of histamine from specialized cells called mast cells. Histamine causes an increase in blood flow, and it changes the walls of small blood vessels to allow fluid and white blood cells to leak out into the damaged tissue. Antihistamines are the medications commonly used to block the inflammatory components of allergic responses. Tissue damage also causes release of a fatty acid called arachidonic acid, which serves as a structural component of cell membranes. The arachidonic acid is quickly converted by enzymes into potent inflammatory substances called prostaglandins. Prostaglandins, in turn, attract cells to clot blood and fight infection, all the while increasing pain and swelling. Aspirin and drugs like ibuprofen give some relief from pain by blocking the conversion of arachidonic acid into these inflammatory substances.

Substances released from injured tissue attract specialized cells of the immune system to come and kill opportunistic bacteria, and to keep watch over the healing process. When initial attempts fail to stop irritation and infection, the body shifts gears and introduces a slightly different set of defensive immune cells. Primary among these cells are the macrophages, a term derived from the Greek for "big eaters." Macrophages can envelope and "eat" bacteria and debris from damaged tissue. The macrophages take up residence in the damaged area and release a stew of powerful chemicals including tumor necrosis factor (TNF), interleukins, prostaglandins, peroxides, and other reactive oxygen species. These substances are necessary to bring infection and injury under control and to initiate healing. However, if sources of inflammation persist and the body's inflammatory response becomes chronic, serious damage can occur.

Doctors have long suspected that chronic inflammation might play a role in Alzheimer's dementia. As early as 1910, only a few years after Alzheimer first described the illness that bears his name, the neuropathologist Oskar Fisher stated his belief that the disease was due to inflammatory effects stimulated by the "foreign material" we now know to be amyloid, which accumulates in the affected brain tissue. The growing consensus among researchers that study Alzheimer's dementia is that Fisher was at least partially correct.

At one time, the brain was thought to be free of immune system cells. However it is now known that cells called glial cells, which reside with neurons in brain tissue, serve a number of different purposes. Glial cells usually perform housekeeping functions in the brain. Some help mop up used neurotransmitters and clean up after neurons die. Others wrap themselves around nerve fibers and form insulation to accelerate and contain electrical impulses. However, when inflammation starts inside the brain, such as from oxidative damage or irritation from collections of amyloid protein, the glial cells can begin to function like macrophages. When amyloid takes up residence in brain tissue, so do the transformed glial cells. Some of the substances released by the transformed glial cells have powerful and, at times, damaging effects on brain tissue. A vicious cycle can begin where inflammation causes an increase in the production of amyloid, and the amyloid in turn serves as an irritant that stimulates further inflammation. Inflammation can also increase the hyperphosphorylation of tau protein that leads to the other classical lesion of Alzheimer's dementia, that is, neurofibrillary tangles.

Chemical markers of inflammation can generally be seen in the blood and cerebrospinal fluid of patients with Alzheimer's. Some, though not all, studies suggest that the concentrations of these inflammatory substances correspond with the severity of the illness. In the well-regarded Framingham Study, nearly seven hundred elderly subjects with normal cognitive function were evaluated. It was found that the subjects with higher blood levels of two specific inflammatory substances, TNF and interleukin-1, were more likely to develop Alzheimer's dementia over the following years. Similar studies have identified two other inflammatory substances in the blood, C-reactive protein (CRP) and interleukin-6, as markers that can help predict the likelihood of developing Alzheimer's dementia. Because inflammation plays an important role in the development of cardiovascular disease, it is not surprising that it also is a risk factor for vascular dementia. High blood levels of interleukin-1, interleukin-6, TNF, CRP, and other common markers of inflammation are generally found in the blood of patients with vascular dementia, and high levels may be useful to predict who is at risk of developing this condition.

Studies of brain tissue from patients with Lewy body dementia also show that immune cells are activated and taking part in inflammatory processes in the brain. This is similar to what is observed in Alzheimer's dementia, although the strength of the inflammatory response may be slightly less severe in Lewy body dementia. Cerebrospinal fluid from patients with frontotemporal dementia also shows increased levels of inflammatory substances, including TNF.

Deposition of amyloid, oxidative stress, and hypoxia can all be direct causes of inflammation in brain tissue. However, it appears that some inflammatory substances, including certain adipocytokines and other substances released into the body from peripheral tissues may also play a role in the inflammatory processes inside the brain. Patients with metabolic syndrome usually have elevated levels of inflammatory substances in their blood. Some of this inflammation is caused by damage from poorly controlled burning of glucose and fat. Prolonged periods of high blood levels of glucose tend to result in the abnormal addition of sugar molecules to proteins, which is a process called glycosylation. Sugar-modified proteins are referred to as advanced glycation endproducts, or more commonly as the acronym AGEs. AGEs are strong stimulators of inflammation in the brain and other tissues. The storage and processing of fats are also poorly controlled in people with high levels of AGEs, and oxidized fats and pro-inflammatory chemicals released from over-burdened visceral fat cells further stimulate inflammation. The increase in inflammation may be one reason why metabolic syndrome is a risk factor for dementia.

For reasons that aren't entirely clear, many individuals suffering major depression also have high blood levels of the same inflammatory cytokines found in metabolic syndrome. Patients with major depression are more than twice as likely than those without depression to have elevated levels of CRP, interleukin-6, and TNF, all of which are markers for inflammation. Insufficient sleep, low blood oxygen from sleep apnea, and poor dietary choices further predispose people to inflammatory processes.

Much of the current interest in inflammation as a factor in dementia arose out of reports from the 1990s that people with long histories of taking non-steroidal anti-inflammatory drugs (NSAIDS) were less likely to develop Alzheimer's dementia. The NSAIDS, which are commonly taken for painful, chronic illnesses such as arthritis, include a number of over-the-counter medications such as ibuprofen, aspirin, naproxen, and others. This class of drugs provides relief from pain and inflammation by preventing the production of prostaglandins.

Laboratory studies have revealed similarities between Lewy body and Alzheimer's dementias in that certain NSAIDs may help prevent the accumulation of abnormal alpha synuclein, which forms the Lewy bodies that characterize both Lewy body dementia and Parkinson's disease. Those initial studies were "test tube" studies and did not involve human subjects. Nonetheless, the results suggest that inflammation plays a role in Lewy body dementia as it does in Alzheimer's, and that medications that reduce inflammation, some as benign and inexpensive as ibuprofen, may help reduce the risk of developing these illnesses.

Although much of the current interest in inflammation was spawned by NSAID reports, controlled studies of the effects of NSAIDs on Alzheimer's have been disappointing. In fact, not all NSAIDs seem to provide protection from the development of Alzheimer's. Negative results have been found in evaluations of naproxen and celecoxib, which is better known as Celebrex. Such findings have led researchers to suspect that the benefits of some NSAIDs may be due to effects other than decrease in inflammation. For example, along with preventing the synthesis of prostaglandins, ibuprofen is also known to reduce production of amyloid, perhaps by reducing the activity of beta-secretase, an enzyme that splices APP into amyloid.

There have been some exciting reports about a medication that can block the effects of TNF, a substance that participates in the inflammatory processes that contribute to Alzheimer's dementia. TNF helps trigger a cascade of events in the brain that eventually results in increases in amyloid plaques and neurofibrillary tangles. It has been reported that injection of etanercept, a drug that blocks the effects of TNF, directly into the cerebrospinal fluid that bathes the brain can produce rapid and dramatic improvements in the cognitive function of patients with Alzheimer's dementia.

HEAD INJURY

I remember as a boy sitting in front of our black and white TV set watching Red Skelton slip into the persona of Cauliflower McPugg, the boxing ring "has been." Dodging and weaving to avoid the imaginary fists flying in the air, Skelton, as McPugg, staggered and mugged for the camera. I laughed myself silly. Unfortunately, this was a time in our culture when tragedies such as dementia, drunk driving, and spousal abuse were not part of our social consciousness.

In fact, a well-known cause of dementia is *dementia pugilistica*, or what has commonly been called being "punch drunk." This is a decline in cognitive function that occurs after repeated head injuries such as prizefighters receive fighting year after year in the boxing ring. The more head punches a fighter receives, the more likely he is to suffer the disorder. In some cases, the presentation of dementia pugilistica is virtually indistinguishable from Alzheimer's dementia. Differences can be noted in the history that led up to the decline in function. Moreover, while neurofibrillary tangles are always present at autopsy in dementia pugilistica, the amyloid plaques that are so prominent in Alzheimer's dementia may not appear until late in the progression of the illness.

The appearance of neurofibrillary tangles may be the first abnormality that appears in the brains of people who suffer repeated head injuries. These tangles of tau protein are frequently seen in retarded individuals with the terrible behavior of head banging, and may even be seen in young football players if they have had more than their share of bad bangs to the head during play. Soccer players can exhibit some of the same changes in brain tissue and cognitive function. It may be a comfort for some to know that this doesn't occur from simply "heading" the ball on repeated occasions, but rather from genuine head injuries sustained during games. This might occur when two players attempt to head the ball, but head each other instead. Another well-known effect of repeated head injury is increased risk for Parkinson's disease. This is likely the cause of the symptoms the great heavyweight boxer Muhammad Ali is now suffering, although it is hard to believe that he was hit enough times to have been placed at risk.

A frightening number of traumatic brain injuries (TBIs) have been sustained by our young soldiers in the Iraq War. Unfortunately, there is growing evidence that TBI is a risk factor for early onset of dementia similar to Alzheimer's dementia. It is now suspected that the so-called shock wave of an explosion does not have to force objects against the head, or even directly reach the head, for brain injury to occur. The high pressures and velocities of shock waves can apparently injure the brain indirectly by forcing waves of pulsations through the arteries into brain tissue. There is even speculation that such explosions can produce electromagnetic radiation that can injure the brain, particularly brains in heads covered by Kevlar helmets rather than the steel helmets used in previous wars. This type of damage can manifest on the microscopic level, and is thus very difficult to appreciate by standards methods such as CAT scans or MRIs. The Department of Defense is investing a great deal of money into investigating the various ways in which explosions injure the brain and how this damage can be avoided or, at least, quickly diagnosed and treated when it does occur.

I feel obligated to add that head injury does not necessarily entail subsequent development of dementia. One of my favorite and most interesting patients, a woman who is now in her eighties, had, about thirty years prior to coming to see me, suffered a catastrophic head injury in a motor vehicle accident. She barely survived her injuries. She had lost the ability to walk, talk, read, and write, and she slowly and laboriously had to relearn the most basic activities of daily living. The injuries she sustained were severe and certain areas of her brain were simply destroyed. This is likely the reason that she is still unable to do many of the things she could do prior to the accident. Although she was a gifted classical pianist, she lost and never recovered her ability to play the piano. In fact, she still struggles to even make sense of music to which she listens. Her very sense of self was disrupted, and she carries a persistent feeling that she has no self. This is particularly tragic when she shows such warmth and humor in her interactions with me. Nonetheless, while some areas of her brain are damaged beyond repair, she exhibits absolutely no indications of any progressive, neurodegenerative processes having been initiated by that trauma to her brain tissue. She reads and loves to discuss with me the latest books on economics and political science. Her memory is probably better than mine. She drives, manages her finances, and cares for herself perfectly well in the home where she lives on her own. Why it is that some people begin to exhibit neurodegenerative changes after a few hard hits in football, whereas others show no such damage even after the very substance of the brain is ripped and shattered is entirely unknown.

BAD TEETH

The elderly are far more likely than the young to suffer tooth loss. It is well known that elderly individuals with dementia have poor dental hygiene habits. Many lose their teeth, and, when teeth remain, there is a greater risk of cavities, gum disease, and further tooth loss than is seen in individuals their age without dementia. In view of these facts, it is not surprising that studies have shown a direct relationship between the number of teeth a person has and the likelihood of having dementia. However, while dementia can increase the risk of dental disease, the opposite might also be true. That is, there is evidence that dental disease, gum disease, and tooth loss may increase the risk of developing dementia.

In a study of comparison between twins, tooth loss before the age of thirty-five was found to be a significant factor in determining the likelihood of later developing Alzheimer's dementia. In a Korean study, elderly subjects who were free of dementia were evaluated for dental health and number of teeth. It was found that those with fewer teeth, particularly if they did not wear dentures, were most likely to develop Alzheimer's dementia in the following years. A European study of elderly nuns found similar results. A perfectly reasonable explanation is that people without teeth are not able to eat properly or absorb necessary nutrients, which would put them at higher risk for dementia. Although this is true to some degree, the relationship between tooth loss and dementia appears to be more complicated than that.

For many years it has been suspected that infections of the teeth and gums can increase the risk of certain types of heart disease. It is known, for example, that the atherosclerotic plaques that build in arteries and cause heart attacks and strokes are often populated by bacteria that live in the mouth. In a study published in the *Archives of Internal Medicine* in 2000, it was found that gum disease is "an important risk factor" for stroke. Any factor that increases the risk of cardiovascular disease and stroke also increases the risk of vascular dementia and, most likely, other forms of dementia.

A particularly disturbing finding is that a spirochete bacteria of the type called *Treponema* is often found in the brains of people diagnosed with Alzheimer's dementia. *Treponema denticola* and related spirochetes are bacteria that normally populate the human mouth. They particularly like plaque that forms on the teeth at the gum line. The numbers of *Treponema denticola* and its relatives dramatically increase in gums that are infected, which is a relatively common condition called gingivitis. It is suspected that these *Treponema* bacteria may find their way from the gums into the trigeminal nerve that supplies the teeth with sensation, migrate up into the brain, and set up housekeeping. Once they are established in the brain, chemical or immunological characteristics of these bacteria appear to trigger neurodegenerative changes that cause dementia. It would not be terribly surprising for a spirochete bacteria to act in this way. Two other even more malign spirochete bacteria, *Treponema pallidum*, which causes syphilis, and *Borrelia burgdorferi*, which causes Lyme disease, are both known to cause similar problems when they infect the brain.

In one of the strangest studies I have ever read, it was shown that simply removing the molars of old rats causes decreases in both spatial memory and the release of the neurotransmitter acetylcholine in certain areas of their cerebral cortex. You might recall that most drugs approved by the

FDA to treat dementia act by increasing the amount of acetylcholine in the brain. This puzzling study would be easy to dismiss were it not for the fact that very similar findings were reported when the molars of aged SAMP8 strain mice were removed. SAMP8 mice are rodents genetically engineered to exhibit changes in the brain and behavior quite similar to those seen in humans with Alzheimer's dementia. Mice that were quaintly described as being in "the molarless condition" had decreases in the amount of acetylcholine in the hippocampus of the brain, something also found in human Alzheimer's patients. Curiously, young SAMP8 mice subjected to "the molarless condition" did not have these reductions in acetylcholine activity. These findings lend an entirely new flavor to the old term "wisdom tooth."

All in all, it seems clear that poor dental hygiene can contribute to dementia by making it difficult to eat and get proper nutrition or by being a source of infection that can spread into the blood or, perhaps, directly into the nervous system from the mouth. It might further contribute through some mysterious and as of yet unexplained mechanism of lowering acetylcholine levels in the brain after teeth are lost.

POOR EDUCATION AND LACK OF MENTAL EXERCISE

One of the most common findings in studies of risk factors for Alzheimer's dementia is that poor education, jobs that do not require much cognitive effort, and a general lack of intellectual stimulation during adult life put people at increased risk for developing dementia at an earlier age and in a more aggressive form. One of the pitfalls of concluding that good educations and intellectually challenging jobs themselves offer protection from dementia is the fact that the people who have them are also likely to have a good income, adequate health care, a healthy diet, and other factors that would independently tend to decrease the risk of dementia. It is also possible that individuals who pursue a good education and seek intellectually challenging jobs are more intelligent from the start. Their high native intelligence, rather than the way they use their minds throughout adult life, may be what reduces their risk for dementia as they age.

In fact, high IQ, even apart from education, appears to have some protective effects against development of Alzheimer's dementia. Nonetheless, college education contributes its own measure of protection from dementia. Benefits of a college education are seen in comparisons of identical twins, when only one of the twins pursued higher education. These benefits are apparent even after income, health care, and overall socioeconomic factors are statistically removed from the equation. In a large study referred to as the East Boston study, it was found that each year of education reduces the risk of Alzheimer's dementia by 17 percent. A study of twins at Duke University found that even apart from a high IQ and a good education, remaining challenged in intellectually stimulating work independently increased the likelihood of avoiding dementia.

There are a number of physiological reasons why intelligence, good education, and exercising the mind might help maintain cognitive function as a person ages. One of the ways in which learning occurs on the neuronal level is by a biochemical process called long-term potentiation, or simply LTP. When neurons fire upon one another repeatedly, dendritic spines that form the chemical connections between the two neurons grow in size and efficiency. This involves the incorporation of special proteins into the dendritic spines, which requires the help of growth factors such as brain-derived neurotrophic factor, or BDNF. The complexity of dendritic branching of nerve cells tends to correspond with their ability to process information. It is possible that people with high IQs are born with unusually high capacity to build and maintain dendritic complexity. In fact, some exceptionally intelligent people have been found to have unique variants of BDNF.

Fortunately, for those of us who aren't born geniuses, pursuing higher education still appears to bring beneficial changes in brain structure and activity. The living brain has tremendous plasticity in dendritic structure and complexity. Stimulation of neurons can rapidly increase branching, mediated in part by BDNF and other growth factors. This occurs in all mammals. For example, studies from the 1960s showed that when rats were raised in interesting, stimulating environments, the neurons in their brains had more extensive dendritic branching than did those of rats raised in plain, featureless cages. Not only does learning make you smarter, but there is evidence that neurons that have been altered by LTP tend to be resistant to the damaging effects of low oxygen levels as well as to the neurotoxic effects of overproduction of the neurotransmitter glutamate. One of the medications approved by the FDA for treatment of dementia, the drug memantine, acts in large part by blocking the neurotoxic effects of glutamate in the brain.

Finally, it is possible that well-educated people may not only better resist damage from neurodegenerative diseases, but even when there is damage, they may be able to use the remaining healthy portions of their brains in more effective manner. A study looked at differences in the brains of Alzheimer's patients with the same degree of cognitive loss, but with some having a history of advanced education and others having little formal education. Amyloid was measured by a new technique in which brain scans pick up signals from a radioactive chemical that binds to and labels amyloid plaques in the brain. The fascinating finding was that while the highly educated patients performed at the same level of cognitive function, they were able to perform at that level despite often suffering more extensive damage from amyloid plaque deposition in their brains.

LACK OF PHYSICAL EXERCISE

Studies show that to avoid dementia, it is important to exercise both the mind and the body. The words of the first-century Roman poet Juvenal, "Mens sana in corpore sano" ("A sound mind in a sound body"), have never grown old. Regular physical exercise improves every aspect of health. It improves cardiovascular condition and lessens the likelihood of metabolic syndrome. It helps reduce obesity and tunes the appetite. It improves sleep and helps reduce stress. There is also compelling evidence that regular physical exercise reduces the risk of dementia.

Physical exercise increases concentrations of BDNF and rates of neurogenesis in the hippocampus. Both of those effects would be expected to offer protection against neurodegenerative processes of dementia. Exercise improves the ability of the brain to deal with oxidative stress, as well as improving the body's regulation of cortisol and other aspects of the stress response. Exciting studies have been performed using mice genetically engineered to carry human genes that produce brain lesions and cognitive losses similar to those of humans with Alzheimer's dementia. Strenuous exercise was shown to both slow down the development of amyloid plaques and to improve learning in those animals.

Human studies lead to similar findings. A Swedish study of identical twins showed that a twin who exercised during middle age was less likely to develop dementia in old age than the twin that did not. Certainly, regular physical exercise can reduce the risk of developing other health problems, such as heart disease and diabetes, that themselves increase the risk of dementia. However, benefits of exercise were seen even after results had been statistically adjusted to remove any good or bad effects of education, diet, smoking, drinking alcohol, and obesity. The strongest effect in that study was seen in preventing vascular dementia, but a protective effect was also seen for Alzheimer's dementia.

All age groups benefit from physical exercise. In one study, people over the age of eight-five who had maintained normal cognitive function were nearly 90 percent more likely to retain cognitive function if they exercised at least four hours per week. Physical exercise on a regular basis even improves the cognitive function of people already diagnosed with Alzheimer's dementia. After three months of daily exercise, participants significantly improved their ability to perform their activities of daily living, such as dressing, personal hygiene, and feeding and toileting themselves.

SMOKING

The number of people who smoke has decreased in the United States over the past fifty years. Current smoking rates are about half of what they were in 1965. However, the rates are still too high, and in some pockets of society, smoking is still quite acceptable. For example, whereas only 5 percent of men and women in the health-care industry are smokers, roughly 40 percent of the mostly men in the construction industry smoke. Overall, about 20 percent, of adults in the United States still smoke.

Smokers don't persist in their habit because they are eager to suffer cardiovascular disease, heart attacks, strokes, and dementia. They smoke because of the pleasurable effects that smoking has on the brain. The nicotine in tobacco smoke has powerful effects on brain activity. Like most addictive substances, nicotine can stimulate the release of the chemical dopamine in parts of the brain that generate feelings of pleasure and reward. Nicotine can also improve certain functions of memory and decision making. Psychiatrists are well aware of the fact that many, if not most, patients with schizophrenia are smokers, because the nicotine helps them organize their thoughts. Unfortunately, the pleasure and the beneficial effects of nicotine on cognitive function are transient, and smokers must continually light up to maintain the desired effects.

The ability of smoking to increase cardiovascular disease is well known. As cardiovascular disease becomes more severe, the risk of all types of dementia increases. The risk of suffering a stroke, and subsequent multi-infarct dementia, increases substantially with the number of cigarettes smoked per day. For smokers, the risk of having a stroke is two or three times greater than for non-smokers. Thankfully, the risk of stroke returns to normal about five years after stopping smoking.

One common effect of smoking that is too often ignored in respect to cognitive function is the incidence of emphysema and chronic bronchitis in lifelong smokers. Lung function usually continues to suffer even after smokers have given up their habit. Chronic obstructive pulmonary disease is the umbrella term for the persistent respiratory problems that smokers and ex-smokers suffer, and it results in chronically low levels of blood oxygen. Not only does low oxygen cause confusion and poor cognitive function, it also compounds inflammation, oxidative stress, and neurodegenerative processes of all kinds, all of which increase the risk of dementia.

Although there is strong evidence that smoking increases the risk of vascular dementia, a direct relationship between smoking and Alzheimer's dementia is less clear. Some studies suggest that smoking more than doubles the risk of Alzheimer's, others show no relationship, whereas a few suggest that smoking may actually decrease the risk of developing the disease. I am not aware of any reports on effects of smoking on the risk of developing Lewy body dementia. However, there is some evidence that smokers enjoy some protection from Parkinson's disease, which is closely related to Lewy body dementia.

There have been a number of explanations for why there has been so much inconsistency in the scientific literature. Some researchers suggest that people who have lived to old age despite having smoked all through adulthood may be a special sort of "hardy survivor." That is, they have an unusually strong constitution that helped them resist both death from cigarette smoking and Alzheimer's dementia. Others suggest that smoking may be a factor in Alzheimer's dementia depending upon whether or not a person carries the APOE4 gene. Data shows that smokers who do develop Alzheimer's dementia tend to develop it at a slightly earlier age than nonsmokers. When a smoker also carries the APOE4 gene, the age of onset is a year or two earlier still. It is possible that some beneficial effects of nicotine on cognitive function may mask or counterbalance the degenerative effects that cigarette smoking might have on the brain. In any case, if you are continuing to smoke out of banking on the possibility that it will spare you from Alzheimer's dementia, you should quit.

ALCOHOL

Moderate intake of alcohol, particularly when taken in the form of red wine, has clearly been found to reduce the risk of dementia. Interestingly, this salutary effect of wine is not limited to human imbibers. I very much enjoyed reading a scientific paper recently published in the prestigious journal *FASEB* that bore the intriguing title, "Moderate Consumption of Cabernet

Sauvignon Attenuates Abeta Neuropathology in a Mouse Model of Alzheimer's Disease."[6]

Opinions vary on the amount of alcohol that is optimal to give protection from dementia. Most studies suggest that people should restrict their intake to no more than a small glass of wine or beer or a shot glass worth of liquor each day. There are also inconsistencies about whether beer, whiskey, and other alcoholic beverages are as helpful as red wine, which contains important antioxidants along with alcohol. In fact, it has been suspected that alcohol itself is not the most important component of red wine in regards to its ability to reduce the risk of cardiovascular disease, metabolic syndrome, and, in turn, dementia. However, a recent study in the *Journal of the American Medical Association* showed that while a daily glass of wine was most effective in reducing the risk of hardening of the arteries and heart attack, moderate consumption of beer and liquor also helped.

The ability of alcoholic beverages to protect against dementia diminishes as intake increases beyond a single small serving a day. Even merely immoderate "social drinkers," who would be shocked at any suspicions that they are alcoholics, can show deficits in abstract thinking and other higher brain function. Heavy drinking has long been known to be a cause of several different forms of dementia. Some dementias related to alcohol abuse are common, particularly vascular dementia. However, some dementias that occur in chronic alcoholics are more exotic.

The dementias caused by heavy drinking are due to varying combinations of the toxic effects of alcohol and the deleterious effects of malnutrition when severe alcoholics go for days replacing eating with drinking alcohol. Although France and Australia both have high per capita intake of alcohol, France has a much lower frequency of alcohol-induced dementia than Australia. This is likely due to the circumstances of the alcohol consumption. In France, the intake of alcohol is primarily in the form of drinking red wine with meals, which would obviously reduce the risk of malnutrition. Nonetheless, there is evidence in the scientific literature that chronic, abusive consumption of large amounts of alcohol, alone and independently of malnutrition, can cause loss of neurons, shrinkage of the brain, and other toxic effects that lead to loss of cognitive function.

Most alcoholics will exhibit some form of cognitive loss after a bout of intoxication. Most will slowly regain normal function over several weeks if

---

6. I personally would have offered the mice a fine Merlot, as it better complements the subtle flavors of the cheese of which they are so fond.

they refrain from alcohol and return to a normal diet and healthful living. In some cases, injections of thiamine or other vitamins are necessary to replenish the brain with essential nutrients and restore function. However, some severe alcoholics will not rebound to normal cognitive function. Instead, they will continue to show varying degrees of cognitive loss due to irreversible alcohol-induced damage to the brain. In some cases, this loss of function is moderate or relatively mild and is referred to as alcohol-related dementia. It is diagnosed by the same criteria as Alzheimer's dementia, except that the patient's history shows that alcoholism has likely played a major role in the development of this loss of cognitive function. There are some indications that abstinence from alcohol, good nutrition, and healthy lifestyle choices can benefit individuals who have been diagnosed with alcohol-related dementia. Of course, Alzheimer's and alcohol-related dementias can occur in the same individual.

Two common forms of alcohol-induced dementia, which are often seen together, are Wernicke's encephalopathy and Korsakoff's syndrome. Both are thought to be due to prolonged periods of heavy drinking in the context of poor nutrition, in particular a lack of the essential vitamin thiamine. Thiamine is one of the B vitamins, and the lack of this vitamin, even in people who are completely abstinent from alcohol, can cause serious and irreversible brain damage. Wernicke's encephalopathy is characterized by confusion and apathy, as well as difficulty with balance and other motor skills, which attests to the fact that the lack of thiamine affects many areas of the brain and a variety of its functions. Korsakoff's syndrome is diagnosed when the patient is no longer able to lay down new memories.

Because of superficial similarities in the two conditions, individuals with Korsakoff's syndrome are often diagnosed as having Alzheimer's disease. However, a long history of severe alcoholism, a history of Wernicke's encephalopathy, appearance of symptoms at a relatively young age, and no family history of early-onset Alzheimer's dementia tends to redirect the diagnosis toward Korsakoff's syndrome. Also, whereas Alzheimer's patients begin to lose social skills and amiability as their illness progresses, patients with Korsakoff's syndrome can remain quite charming and sociable. Lacking the ability to remember recent events, they can sometimes weave elaborate tales about the circumstances that brought them to the hospital or care facility where their illness has forced them to be placed. This making up of stories to explain away circumstances in a socially acceptable fashion is called confabulation. Confabulation is far more common in Korsakoff's syndrome than in Alzheimer's dementia.

Marchiafava-Bignami disease is an unusual dementing illness that was first described in 1903 in Italian men who spent their lives overindulging in red wine. There have only been a few hundred recorded cases. The illness is unlikely to be caused entirely by the red wine itself, as a few cases have been seen in patients who did not use alcohol of any type. Nonetheless, its appearance among red wine drinkers speaks to the fact that even this generally beneficial substance should be consumed with moderation. Marchiafava-Bignami disease often presents as dementia with mood changes, muscle spasticity, difficulty walking, and seizures. In these respects, the condition can resemble Binswanger's disease. One of the major findings in scanning the brains of sufferers of Marchiafava-Bignami disease by MRI is degeneration of the corpus callosum, which is the bridge of white matter containing nerve fibers that connect the two sides of the brain. This does not occur in Binswanger's disease or other forms of dementia. Marchiafava-Bignami disease invariably progresses to a bad conclusion.

Alcohol can either reduce or increase the risk of various types of dementia, depending upon the amount and type of alcoholic beverage an individual consumes, and the degree to which intemperate drinking replaces a healthy diet. All in all, the most prudent advice that I have heard about consuming alcohol is that people who drink heavily should be told to stop, people who drink in moderation should be allowed to continue to do so, and people who do not drink should not be encouraged to start. As with smoking, there is evidence that presence of the APOE4 gene can increase the risk of Alzheimer's dementia in people who are heavy drinkers. In people who carry the APOE4 gene, the extra combination of smoking and heavy drinking adds up to a serious triple threat that decreases the age of onset of Alzheimer's dementia from an average of seventy-seven down to sixty-eight, with no other major risk factors.

MARIJUANA

It has been estimated that as many as seven million people in the United States smoke marijuana on at least a weekly basis. There are conflicting opinions about what, if any, role marijuana may have in causing loss of cognitive function or dementia. Marijuana causes its unique effects on the mind and brain by mimicking a family of substances in the brain called "endocannabinoids." The prefix "endo" refers to the substance being endogenous or natural to the brain, and it is the same prefix in the word "endorphins," which are endogenous morphine-like molecules in brain tissue.

Endocannabinoids are important chemical messengers in the brain. They are involved in the processing of anxiety and fear responses, which may be part of what makes them pleasurable for some people.

There are inconsistencies in the scientific literature about the role played by endocannabinoids in human cognitive function. Endocannabinoid receptor (CB-1) knock-out mice, that is, mice that have had their genetic codes manipulated so that they do not produce receptors for endocannabinoids, exhibit a number of cognitive abnormalities. Curiously, CB-1 knock-out mice have enhancement of some memory functions, which suggests that endocannabinoids may slow down or prevent some types of learning. It might at first seem odd that a natural substance in the brain would impair learning. However, the usefulness of such a mechanism could be in a phenomenon called extinction, which is an active form of forgetting things that are no longer useful or relevant.

Those who smoke marijuana are not surprised to learn that being "stoned" on the drug causes deficits in attention, memory, judgment, speed of cognitive processing, time estimation, and dexterity. However, heavy users of marijuana show such deficits even after four weeks of abstaining from the drug. There are also reports of reduction in the activity of the frontal lobes in chronic marijuana smokers. Electrical activity, as seen in electroencephalograms, or brain wave studies, slows down in the brains of heavy marijuana users. Blood flow to the brain also tends to be reduced. Those reductions persist for up to a month after quitting. Animal studies have shown that exposure to high levels of marijuana decreases the ability of neurons in the brain to lay down memories. This effect is thought to be caused by THC, the component of marijuana that is also thought to be responsible for the "high" produced by the drug.

The above findings would not seem to bode well for the maintenance of normal cognitive function in marijuana smokers. However, many studies show that marijuana-related abnormalities in brain activity and function reverse with time. Long-term use of marijuana has no effect on the size of the hippocampus, an area of the brain required for the making and storage of new memories. This is the area of the brain that is most seriously damaged in Alzheimer's dementia. A study performed at Boston University compared the intelligence test scores of pairs of identical twins in which only one of the twins was a chronic, long-term marijuana smoker. No significant differences in intelligence were found between the marijuana smoking and abstaining twins. Several studies, including a large study performed at Johns Hopkins University, have shown that heavy users of marijuana are no more likely than non-users to develop

Alzheimer's or other forms of dementia. There are some differing reports. One study found that long-term, heavy smokers of marijuana, with subjects smoking at least five joints a day for an average of twenty years, did show shrinking of the hippocampus as well as loss of cognitive function. I do wonder if some of the loss of brain tissue and cognitive function was due to the marijuana itself or to being too intoxicated to go out and be active and stimulated by new experiences in the world. In any case, moderation is again the most prudent approach for people who smoke marijuana. Abstainers should probably not be advised to start, unless compelling reasons emerge, such as pain or nausea from a new medical problem.

Of particular interest are recent findings that some components of marijuana may actually help prevent the development of Alzheimer's dementia. As is generally the case with herbal preparations, marijuana contains many chemicals that are similar in structure but quite different in effects. THC, which causes the intoxicating effect of marijuana, has also been found to be a powerful inhibitor of an enzyme called acetylcholinesterase, which is the same mechanism of action of Aricept and several other drugs prescribed to treat Alzheimer's dementia. THC also appears to slow down production of amyloid, which accumulates as neuritic plaques in the brain tissue of Alzheimer's patients. Cannabidiol, another substance in marijuana, does not cause intoxication. However, it does help prevent the hyperphosphorylation of tau protein that leads to the formation of neurofibrillary tangles in Alzheimer's dementia. It may also protect the brain from the neurodegenerative effects of amyloid. However, in view of the fact that simply smoking marijuana doesn't offer any protection from developing Alzheimer's dementia, and may even contribute to cognitive loss in some individuals, it is reasonable to assume that high doses of specific, purified components of marijuana would be necessary to achieve any benefit. This is an active area of research.

BACTERIAL AND VIRAL CAUSES OF DEMENTIA

Dementia is generally thought to arise from a combination of genetic predisposition and unhealthy lifestyle choices. However, there is a surprisingly large and growing literature suggesting that bacterial and viral infections may contribute to the development of some dementias, including Alzheimer's. People with Alzheimer's dementia are far more likely than non-demented people of the same age to have evidence of infection by a bacteria called *Chlamydia pneumoniae*.[7] Chlamydial infection is also seen to be a risk factor for heart disease; however, the association between this bacteria and the risk of vascular dementia is less clear.

Chlamydia pneumoniae has an affinity for brain cells, and in patients with Alzheimer's dementia, it is found in high concentrations in areas of the brain where plaques and tangles appear. This suggests that infection by the bacteria may stimulate inflammatory processes that exacerbate the neurodegenerative effects of Alzheimer's. Scientists are currently studying whether treating or vaccinating against chlamydial infection can reduce the risk of dementia or improve symptoms in patients diagnosed with Alzheimer's.

Syphilis, a sexually transmitted disease caused by the spirochete bacteria *Treponema pallidum*, has long been known to cause a particularly severe form of dementia in its later stages. Lyme disease, which is caused by a related spirochete bacteria, *Borrelia burgdorferi*, can also cause cognitive disturbances if not diagnosed and treated in timely fashion. Both of these bacteria can alter amyloid and tau protein in the brain and cause symptoms that can be easily confused with Alzheimer's dementia. Unlike *Chlamydia pneumoniae*, neither bacteria is thought to be a cause of true Alzheimer's dementia. Thankfully, dementia caused by syphilis has become rare in the past twenty years. The incidence of Lyme disease, however, has been on the rise, and cognitive and psychiatric changes due to this infective illness may be underdiagnosed. As I've noted previously, some spirochetes related to the ones that cause syphilis and Lyme disease may contribute to dementia in people with decayed teeth and gum infections.

The common bacteria *Helicobacter pylori* is recently coming into focus as a contributing factor in a variety of human health problems. The physician and scientist Dr. Barry Marshall shared the Nobel Prize for Medicine with Dr. Robin Warren in 2005 for establishing the fact that most cases of stomach ulcers are caused not by worry and stress, but rather by infection of the stomach lining with *Helicobacter pylori*. In the initial stages of his research, the intrepid Marshall proved his theory by drinking a flask of the bacteria and later developing ulcers, as he had predicted.

There are a number of studies showing that people with dementia are more likely than not to have had a history of gastric infection by *Helicobacter pylori*. One study has shown that patients diagnosed with Alzheimer's dementia are nearly twice as likely to be positive for *Helicobacter*

---

7. *Chlamydia pneumoniae* is different from a related bacteria called *Chlamydia trachomatis*, which is the variety of chlamydia responsible for several common sexually transmitted diseases.

pylori than people of their age without this dementia. The apparent relationship between *Helicobacter pylori* and dementia may simply be due to decreases in absorption of vitamin B_{12} that may persist after the bacteria causes damage to the stomach lining. However, a recent study suggests that the risk of Alzheimer's dementia is increased in people positive for infection with *Helicobacter pylori* even when there is no evidence of damage to the stomach lining or low levels of vitamin B_{12}.

An intriguing connection between bacteria and risk for developing dementia comes from evidence that intestinal bacteria can affect obesity in hitherto unexpected ways. The balance between two types of bacteria indigenous to the human intestine, *Firmicutes* and *Bacteroidetes*, can change the way the gut absorbs calories and thereby alter the risk of becoming obese. Obese people have a higher proportion of *Firmicutes* bacteria in their gut than do lean people. In turn, *Firmicutes* colonization appears to stimulate uptake and deposition of fat in the adipocytes, as well as to increase inflammation and insulin resistance. Thus *Firmicutes* may participate in an upward spiral into obesity and metabolic syndrome. Gut bacteria may be brought into healthier balance by improving the diet, supplementing with "probiotics," or including fermented products such as yogurt in the diet. This may be particularly important after oral antibiotic treatments for infections.

Several viruses have also been associated with dementias. The common virus herpes simplex type 1 can cause abnormalities in amyloid and tau protein in the brain and may stimulate pathological deposition of these proteins as is seen in Alzheimer's dementia. Herpes simplex infection may be a risk factor for the development of Alzheimer's dementia, particularly in people who carry the APOE4 gene. The APOE4 may help the virus enter the brain, which is not its usual site of infection. Herpes simplex type 1 is related to, but not the same as, herpes simplex type 2, which is the virus responsible for the well-known sexually transmitted disease that is commonly referred to as genital herpes. Another virus similar to herpes simplex, cytomegalovirus, has been associated with vascular dementia.

The human immunodeficiency virus (HIV), which causes acquired immunodeficiency syndrome (AIDS), may also cause a type of dementia in some patients suffering that illness. Both the cognitive and neurodegenerative changes seen in HIV-induced dementia can be very similar to those of Alzheimer's dementia, including abnormalities in the processing of tau and amyloid protein. I have had the sad experience of seeing young men in their forties exhibit signs of dementia due to HIV.

Antibodies to the Epstein-Barr virus have been found to react with certain forms of the protein alpha-synuclein in the human brain. In other words, antibodies produced by the body to fight off the Epstein-Barr virus may also inadvertently attack alpha-synuclein in the brain. Alpha-synuclein is one of the proteins that is abnormally processed in Parkinson's disease and Lewy body dementia. It remains to be determined whether infection by Epstein-Barr virus increases the risk of Lewy body dementia.

The rare, but devastating dementing illness Creutzfeldt-Jakob disease is caused by a peculiar agent of infection called a prion. A prion is not even as complex as a virus, but rather it is an abnormal form of protein that initiates a pathological process of protein crystallization in the brain. This illness can evolve for no obvious reason in certain unlucky individuals. It can also be acquired in an infective fashion when the prion is consumed in meat from cattle suffering mad cow disease, which is merely the bovine form of Creutzfeldt-Jakob Disease. At one time, cannibalistic natives of Borneo were vulnerable to a similar illness called Kuru, which they contracted by eating the infected brains of vanquished enemies.[8] After cannibalism was wiped out in that area at the end of the twentieth century, Kuru was eliminated as well.

There are some fascinating reports about a prion brain disease similar to Creutzfeldt-Jakob disease observed in some people from Kentucky that is believed to be caused by eating improperly cooked, infected squirrel brains.[9] In fact, there may be many forms of prion diseases in the animal kingdom that affect brain tissue. It is not known to what degree humans are susceptible.

ENVIRONMENTAL CAUSES

It has long been suspected that factors in the environment may contribute to the development of dementia. Among these environmental factors are low-frequency electromagnetic radiation, aluminum, heavy metals, pes-

---

8. The name of the brain disease Kuru can easily be confused with the equally dreadful, yet even more bizarre culture-bound psychosis known as Koro. Koro, which is rarely seen outside of the Orient, is the psychotic delusion that one's penis is shrinking and withdrawing back into the body. The psychosis tends to include the delusion that if the penis withdraws completely, the sufferer will die. As absurd as this delusion may seem, some cultures take it quite seriously, to the point of men forming alliances with other men who promise, should the need arise, to grab the victim's penis, pull on it, and thus prevent it from withdrawing back into the body to kill the unfortunate fellow. Epidemics of Koro in villages in Southeast Asia have been reported in the literature.

9. Of course, this presumes that there is a *proper* way to cook squirrel brains, which I suspect is not true.

ticides, air pollution, water pollution, and other forms of contamination. Most of these are avoidable, although some of these are so prevalent in modern society that escape from them may require some effort.

Over the past twenty-five years, evidence has accumulated to conclude that exposure to extremely low-frequency electromagnetic fields (ELF-EMF) can increase the risk of Alzheimer's dementia. Laboratory studies have shown that exposure of human brain cells to ELF-EMF increases their production of forms of amyloid protein that are found in the brains of patients with Alzheimer's. Epidemiological studies have shown that workers exposed to ELF-EMF in certain high-risk occupations, such as power plant employees, arc welders, and electrical engineers, have increased rates of Alzheimer's dementia.

Unfortunately, sources of exposure to ELF-EMF in modern society are everywhere. Among the many common devices and objects that emit ELF-EMF are cell phones, high voltage electrical transmission lines, electric blankets, hair dryers, and any other electrical device in which there is flow of electrical current, an electrical motor, or a heating coil. The type, intensity, and duration of exposure necessary to increase the risk of Alzheimer's dementia is unclear. There has been a great deal of publicity in the media about a possible connection between cell phone use and brain tumors. However, little or nothing has been said about effects of cell phones on the risk of Alzheimer's dementia. Nonetheless, if the threat of tumors with cell phones is genuine, and many credible scientists see the data as ominous, then there should be concern about Alzheimer's as well.

Environmental exposures to heavy metals, such as lead and mercury, have also been suspected of contributing to dementia. The Latin word for lead is "plumbum," and from it we derive the word "plumber." Ancient Roman plumbers commonly used lead while plying their craft, because the soft, heavy metal was so easily formed into pipe or pounded flat into sheets to form impervious linings for cisterns. It has been suggested by some historians that lead poisoning, with its ability to addle the mind and brain, contributed to the decline and fall of the Roman Empire. While that theory remains controversial, historical records show that the Romans themselves were well aware of the dangers of lead, and when possible they avoided its use.

In the recent past, exposure to lead has come primarily through the use of this metal as an additive in paint and gasoline. The environmental risks of lead were eventually recognized and, thankfully, these dangerous practices were phased out in the 1980s. Exposure to lead has consequently dropped dramatically over the past twenty-five years, and lead toxicity is now much less of a concern. Unfortunately, problems of lead toxicity are not entirely gone.

Studies as recent as 2005 have shown that poorer people living in inner cities, particularly in the Northeastern urban areas of the United States, are still at risk for having elevated blood levels of lead. Some people are still being exposed to dangerous levels of lead at the workplace. Not surprisingly, miners of lead ore and people who work as lead smelters are often found to have high levels of lead in their blood. Construction workers, particularly those who renovate old buildings, can also be exposed to lead. Those who work in the glass industry or manufacture storage batteries are at risk of exposure. Certain hobbies, such as working with ceramics or stained glass, can also increase the risk of toxic blood levels of lead.

Lead can also still exist in unsafe levels in drinking water. Several years ago, *The Washington Post* published a report in which they reviewed data collected by the Environmental Protection Agency. That data, some of it as recent as the year 2000, identified 274 different municipal water systems across the United States that supplied water with unsafe concentrations of lead. Those systems served over 11.5 million people and put them at risk of lead toxicity. Another ominous fact is that the United States Center for Disease Control has recently found that blood lead levels necessary to adversely affect the brain are much lower than were once thought.

The treatment for severe lead poisoning is chelation therapy. Chelators, molecules that take their name from the Greek word for "claw," are shaped in such a way that they can grab lead atoms and escort them out of the body. However, chelation therapy has its own dangers, and the favored treatment for milder lead toxicity is simply to remove the source of lead contamination and wait for blood levels to decrease. However, a rather sobering study of laboratory monkeys has shown that exposure to lead very early in life, even in infancy, can trigger long-lasting changes in the brain that years later can contribute to Alzheimer's dementia. These changes include damage to neuronal DNA and increases in deposition of amyloid in the frontal cortex. Thus, in some cases, lowering blood lead levels may have limited benefits, as the damage may already have been done. Nonetheless, it is wise to reduce exposure to this toxic metal. Exposure to lead in adulthood increases the expression of amyloid precursor protein, and makes the sticky 1-42 of amyloid even stickier and more likely to accumulate as plaque. Lead increases oxidative stress, causes mitochondrial damage, and triggers inflammation in brain tissue. Lead inhibits the birth of new neurons by neurogenesis, and it interferes with the process of long-term potentiation that is necessary for the laying down of memories. A recent Japanese study has found that a relatively rare form of frontotemporal dementia in humans, called diffuse neurofibrillary tangles with calcification, or alternatively Kosaka-Shibayama disease, is likely to be caused by chronic exposure to lead.

Exposure to mercury causes many of the same adverse effects as lead. Mercury has specifically been found to stimulate formation of the insoluble beta amyloid found in Alzheimer's. A controversial question is whether or not the mercury-containing amalgam that dentists have long used to fill cavities in teeth might contribute to Alzheimer's dementia or other neurodegenerative diseases, such as multiple sclerosis or Parkinson's disease. A report in a German neurological journal stated that mercury levels can be two to ten times higher in the brain tissue of people who have amalgam fillings than in tissue of those who don't. Nonetheless, there is no solid evidence in the research literature to support the conclusion that amalgam fillings increase the risk of Alzheimer's dementia.

High intake of aluminum has been associated with Alzheimer's dementia. However, the clearest examples of aluminum causing dementia are from the past when it was inadvertently introduced into the bloodstream in patients on dialysis treatment for kidney failure. That problem was corrected long ago, and aluminum-induced dementia is now difficult to find. Thankfully, aluminum is very poorly absorbed from the gut. Thus, even large amounts of aluminum in the diet may not be of great concern. In the United States, aluminum is used as a food additive, primarily in the form of sodium silicoaluminate or sodium aluminophosphate, to prevent caking of powders in prepared foods. A breakfast of pancakes or waffles from a dry mix may contain as much as 180 mg of aluminum. People taking antacids, which often contain aluminum hydroxide, can consume ten times that amount each day. It is a relief to note that beverages from aluminum cans are almost certainly not significant sources of aluminum. A soft drink from inside an aluminum can usually contains only about 0.5 mg of aluminum, even if it has sat on the shelf for months.

There has long been a controversy as to whether fluoride, primarily from fluoridation of drinking water, plays any role in Alzheimer's dementia. There are studies using laboratory rats showing that chronic exposure to 1 ppm fluoride in drinking water for one year led to plaques and tangles in the rats' brains quite similar to those seen in the brain tissue of patients with Alzheimer's. However, given that fluoride has been added to the water supply of many if not most American cities since the 1940s, one would think that we would have a clearer sense of whether or not it exacerbates the illness in humans. Curiously, the only epidemiological study of fluoride has suggested that fluoride in drinking water may actually *reduce* the risk of Alzheimer's.

Part of the uncertainty about the effects of fluoride on Alzheimer's dementia may arise from the fact that fluoride interacts with aluminum, and can either increase or diminish the impact that aluminum might have on the body. It is known, for example, that fluoride and aluminum compete for absorption in the gut, thus fluoride in the drinking water might reduce the risk of Alzheimer's dementia by preventing absorption of aluminum into the bloodstream. On the other hand, there is also evidence that when an individual cooks using aluminum pots and pans, fluoride in the cook water can increase the amount of aluminum that leaches out of the pan and into the food. Although various groups have long and bitterly complained about fluoride in the water supply, it is worth noting that many mouthwashes and toothpastes have concentrations of fluoride hundreds of times higher than those seen in fluoridated drinking water.

A more recently recognized risk factor is bisphenol A, or BPA. BPA is used in the manufacturing of plastics, and it is found in many food and drink containers. It is sometimes in products where you would not expect it. For example, while you might think the tin can containing the soup you are about to eat is made entirely from metal, it is likely to be lined with a film of plastic that has been made with BPA. This substance contaminates an astonishing variety of foods. The 2003–2004 National Health and Nutrition Examination Survey conducted by the Centers for Disease Control and Prevention found detectable levels of BPA in 93 percent of 2,517 urine samples from people six years and older in age. Scientists have long known that BPA can cause damage in rat brains. A greater concern is a recent report that monkey brains, which are even more similar to our own, are also damaged by BPA. BPA and several other similar chemicals in plastics also have properties similar to estrogen in the mammalian body. In view of unresolved issues as to what effects estrogens have on the brain and the development of dementia, the finding of estrogenic effects of these substances is disturbing.

Toxins that we are exposed to in food and water can also be taken in from the air we breathe. Over the past ten years or so, a troubling, but not altogether surprising, series of studies on the effects of air pollution on dementia has been performed by Dr. Calderón-Garcidueñas at the Instituto Nacional de Pediatría, in Mexico City. Mexico City has some of the most highly polluted air in the world. In some of his initial studies, Calderón-Garcidueñas found that dogs living in Mexico City that were forced to breathe the polluted air tended to develop inflammation, plaques, and tangles in their brains similar to those found in human patients with Alzheimer's dementia. He then performed autopsies on people who had lived in Mexico City and other areas with high levels of air pollution and found that the degree of accumulation of amyloid and signs of inflammation in their brain tissue were higher than those found in the brains of individuals who had lived in areas with cleaner air. A particularly concerning finding was that these changes in brain tissue suggestive of early stages of Alzheimer's dementia could be observed not only in elderly people, but also in young adults and children. Along with accumulation of amyloid, Calderón-Garcidueñas also found abnormal deposits of alpha-synuclein, which is the type of lesion seen in Parkinson's disease and Lewy body dementia.

An underappreciated source of environmental health risks is radon. Radon is a radioactive gas that is found in varying degrees in most regions of the United States. There are relatively high concentrations of radon in the Appalachian Mountain states, the Sierra Nevada Mountain areas of California, and in many of the Northern Plains states. The primary source of radon gas is slow leaks from local rock and soil. Radon gas is heavier than air, so it tends to collect in low areas of houses, particularly in basements. A high concentration of radon in the air is known to be a major risk factor for lung cancer. It is thought to play a role in the development of 10 to 15 percent of lung cancers in the United States. Of significant concern are reports that radon and, more specifically, radioactive byproducts of exposure to radon, tend to accumulate in specific areas of the brain. Among the areas of the brain most affected by radon are the hippocampus, temporal lobes, and frontal lobes. Exposure to radon gas adversely affects brain tissue. One author stated that radon exposure "dramatically" increased rates of cell loss and deposition of amyloid in the same areas of the brain where cell loss, amyloid plaques, and neurofibrillary tangles are seen in patients with Alzheimer's dementia. Further study is needed to determine if a high radon level is yet another risk factor for dementia. However, given the proven effects of radon on lung cancer, it would be wise to test for radon levels in high risk parts of the country and to take appropriate measures as needed. Your local county health department should have information to give you of what the risk in your area may be.

Other aspects of modern life can unexpectedly contribute to the risk of dementia. For example, it has been reported that many anesthetics inhaled by patients undergoing surgery can increase the generation of amyloid protein in brain tissue. Some studies have indeed suggested that having had general anesthesia can increase the risk of Alzheimer's dementia. Individuals in certain occupations are at higher risk than others for developing Alzheimer's dementia. Hairdressers are among the people at enhanced risk. This may be due to constantly being around hair dryers and the relatively high amount of ELF-EMF they generate. People who have frequent job exposures to pesticides and organic solvents are at increased risk. For some professions, their somewhat higher statistical risk for Alzheimer's is very difficult to explain. For example, in some studies, such groups have included bank tellers and clergyman. No one knows why this is the case.

6

VITAMINS, HERBS, AND
NUTRACEUTICALS

In this chapter, I will discuss some interesting and potentially useful herbs, vitamins, and nutraceuticals. Some I recommend to my own patients, whereas others are simply prominent enough in the public eye that they deserve to be discussed and critiqued. At the current state of the art of treating dementia, there is still no way to reverse the damage caused by the underlying neurodegenerative processes once they have begun. Even with the most potent and expensive medications that are approved by the FDA to treat dementia, the best result one should hope for is only a slowing down, not an arrest or reversal of the process. With this in mind, I must emphasize that none of the herbs, vitamins, and nutraceuticals I am going to discuss should be seen as cures for dementia, nor even as treatments that can with any certainty slow its progression. In fact, some of these substances have been scientifically evaluated as treatments for dementia and found to be ineffective in changing the course of dementia once it has started.

The supplements I will discuss do not erase ill effects of dietary indiscretions, nor do they replace exercise, stress reduction, and other good lifestyle choices. There are reasons to believe, however, that the effects of many of these substances can help prevent the initiation, and perhaps the progression, of some of the pathological processes that lead to dementia. This would be expected to be most effective if they were consumed on a regular basis in one's forties or fifties, when these processes tend to begin. Among the ways these substances may help prevent dementia are antioxidant and anti-inflammatory effects, stimulation of neuron growth factors such as BDNF, reduction of the synthesis and accumulation of sticky beta amyloid protein, enhancement of acetylcholine activity, and decrease in the manifestations of metabolic syndrome, which would include stabilization of blood sugar levels, improvement in levels of serum cholesterol and other lipids, normalization of blood pressure, and decreases in insulin resistance.

ACETYL-CARNITINE

Acetyl-carnitine is a natural substance in the body. It is formed in cells by the enzymatic addition of an "acetyl" group to the amino acid carnitine. Carnitine serves an important role in the ability of cells to burn fat. It carries fat molecules across the walls of the mitochondria, where they are oxidized and turned into energy. On its return trip from inside the mitochondria, it brings back acetyl groups that the cell uses to synthesize other molecules it needs, including the neurotransmitter acetylcholine, which plays such an important role in dementia. Although carnitine is primarily involved in fat metabolism, its activities affect all the other aspects of energy metabolism in the cell, including the burning of carbohydrate. In this way it can be linked to glucose metabolism, insulin, and metabolic syndrome.

The major difference between acetyl-carnitine and carnitine is that acetyl-carnitine is more easily absorbed from the gut and more readily crosses the fatty barrier between the blood and the brain. Thus, as a supplement, acetyl-carnitine has certain advantages. Because most of us eat meat, which is rich in carnitine, most of us get a constant supply of this amino acid–like substance in our diet. Moreover, all of us make carnitine and acetyl-carnitine in our bodies. Thus, it is not entirely clear if it is necessary to supplement the diets of healthy people with carnitine or acetyl-carnitine. However, it has been found that carnitine levels decrease significantly as we age.

Recent evidence suggests that acetyl-carnitine may offer some protection from oxidative damage, and this protection may even extend to the brain. A study has found that treating rat brain cells with acetyl-carnitine decreases the damage caused by beta amyloid. It also decreases the likelihood of those cells dying by apoptosis. Giving acetyl-carnitine to very old rats lowers the concentrations of cholesterol and triglycerides in their blood. Recent studies have found that acetyl-carnitine can help prevent decreases in sensitivity to insulin caused by inflammatory substances in the body. These effects would help the body resist the development of dementia by reducing the risk of metabolic syndrome, heart disease, and diabetes. No such studies have been performed in healthy elderly human beings.

There is compelling evidence that 1.5 to 3 grams a day of acetyl-carnitine can improve the cognitive function of individuals in the milder, early stages of Alzheimer's disease. It is not clear if acetyl-carnitine improves cognition by improving mitochondrial activity in the brain or by making more acetyl groups available to be used in the synthesis of the neurotransmitter acetylcholine in the brain. Acetylcholine levels are decreased in many forms of dementia, and most of drugs used for treatment of Alzheimer's disease increase the availability of acetylcholine by preventing its enzymatic destruction in the brain. As a psychiatrist, I am particularly interested in a number of recent reports that acetyl-carnitine can be helpful in the treatment of depression in elderly patients.

Overall, it can be safely stated that there is evidence from both human and animal studies that carnitine, or its more readily absorbed form, acetyl-carnitine, can to some degree improve glucose tolerance, insulin sensitivity, serum lipids, and cognitive function. It may also provide some protection from oxidative damage. Depression and fatigue can be improved. Studies of the effects of acetyl-carnitine on the human brain are ongoing. However, the Cochrane reviewers, a very well-respected English research group dedicated to studying and publishing reports on various medical treatments, has stated that acetyl-carnitine is likely to prove to be an important therapeutic agent.

Acetyl-carnitine is a natural substance with little likelihood of producing adverse effects. There have been reports of high doses of acetyl-carnitine causing seizures in rats; however, I am not aware of any such reports in humans when taken in typical doses of 500 milligrams to 2 grams a day. It is one of the supplements that I take on a daily basis, and I do not hesitate to recommend it.

ALPHA-LIPOIC ACID

Alpha-lipoic acid is another natural substance in the human body. We synthesize our own alpha-lipoic acid in the liver and other tissues. We also obtain some in our diet, primarily from organ meats. However, some researchers suspect that our synthesis and consumption of alpha-lipoic acid are barely adequate and so supplementation is useful.

Alpha-lipoic acid is a potent antioxidant molecule. As an antioxidant, it reduces a variety of sources of oxidative stress in the body. It is also known to reactivate vitamins E and C after they have been used as antioxidants. Whereas vitamin E is soluble in fat and vitamin C is soluble in water, alpha-lipoic acid is soluble in both fat and water. Thus, it has full access to all tissues of the body, including the brain.

Alpha-lipoic acid is also known to be an important co-factor in the burning of glucose in the mitochondria, the energy-producing factories inside every cell. However, the effects of alpha-lipoic acid on glucose metabolism may be more complicated than that. Studies have suggested that alpha-lipoic acid may mimic some of the effects that insulin has on cells in the body. Like insulin, it tells the liver to stop secreting glucose into the blood and increases uptake of glucose from the blood by stimulating special glucose transport mechanisms in cell membranes. Alpha-lipoic acid also reduces serum triglyceride levels in laboratory rats, as would be expected of a substance that mimics or enhances the effects of insulin. It has been found that alpha-lipoic acid significantly improves insulin sensitivity in diabetic patients.

Alpha-lipoic acid has been found to reduce the ability of the troublesome chemical messenger of fat cells and the immune system, tumor necrosis factor alpha (TNF-alpha), to activate nuclear factor-kappaB (NF-κB). NF-κB is a chemical switch that initiates some important inflammatory processes. It sets into motion the production of a variety of substances that promote metabolic syndrome. Thus alpha-lipoic acid acts to dampen the oxidative damage, inflammation, weight gain, and insulin resistance that drive metabolic syndrome and neurodegenerative processes in the brain that lead to dementia.

In the brain, alpha-lipoic acid can help prevent damage from oxidation, as well as protect it from the toxic, inflammatory effects of beta amyloid. When given to old mice genetically altered to overproduce beta amyloid in their brains, alpha-lipoic acid reduced evidence of oxidative damage and, more importantly, improved memory functions. The combination of alpha-lipoic acid and acetyl-carnitine has been found to be particularly potent in animal studies. In a study in human patients with Alzheimer's dementia, 600 mg per day of alpha-lipoic acid dramatically slowed deterioration of cognitive function over the four years the study took place.

The insulin-enhancing, antioxidant, and anti-inflammatory effects of alpha-lipoic acid would appear to make it a very useful substance. Moreover, there appears to be little if any toxicity of the substance. Because alpha-lipoic acid competes with the B vitamins biotin and pantothenic acid for uptake into cells, it has been suggested that supplementation with alpha-lipoic acid should also include supplementation with the B-complex of vitamins.

As a word of warning, taking alpha-lipoic acid will cause your urine to have the same peculiar, sulfurous smell that it gets when you eat asparagus.

ASHWAGANDHA

Ashwagandha is a fascinating herb that has been used in traditional folk medicines in the Middle East and in the sophisticated Hindu Ayurvedic system of medicine for thousands of years. Ashwagandha has been used to treat a wide spectrum of medical problems that have included inflammation, fatigue, mood disorders, sexual problems, and insomnia. It has been considered to act generally as a tonic for all manners of weakness and ill health.

The scientific name for the ashwagandha plant is *Withania somnifera*, and references to this plant in western literature began to appear in the early 1950s. A number of biologically active substances, known as withanolides, can be extracted from ashwagandha. The withanolides are molecules similar in structure to steroids, and dozens of different varieties of withanolides have been identified in crude extracts of plant material. Western studies have suggested that most of the medicinal effects of ashwagandha are due to the actions of two of these withanolides, withaferin A and withanolide D. However, as is often the case in herbal preparations, other substances in the plant may contribute subtle but important effects in people taking the herb as treatment for their medical problems. Laboratory studies, historical references, and anecdotal evidence all point to the possibility that ashwagandha and the withanolides may offer benefits in the treatment and prevention of dementia.

Scientific studies have revealed some very impressive effects of ashwagandha on the brain and body. In test tube studies, ashwagandha was found to reduce the production of the advanced glycation endproducts (AGEs) in tissue from diabetic rats. AGEs stimulate inflammation and accelerate the neurodegenerative processes in Alzheimer's dementia. Ashwagandha also blocks the effects of the cellular trigger of inflammation NF-κB and contains antioxidants to protect the brain from oxidative stress. Several studies show that withanolides can inhibit both acetylcholinesterase and butyrylcholinesterase (enzymes that break down acetylcholine), albeit with less potency than do the cholinesterase inhibitors that are prescribed to treat dementia. Of particular interest are studies showing that treatment with ashwagandha can stimulate neurons to grow the dendritic branches they use to communicate with each other and to regenerate dendrites that have been damaged by exposure to amyloid.

When laboratory rats were treated with ashwagandha or specific extracts of the plant, they were far better able to withstand stressful conditions. Stressors that included cold temperature, low oxygen, sleep deprivation, and mild but unpredictable electrical foot shocks caused high levels of stress hormones, high blood sugar, oxidative damage, and learning deficits. All of these adverse effects were reduced by ashwagandha. Rats subjected to severe and prolonged stress also suffer loss of neurons in an area of the brain called the hippocampus. When rats are treated with ashwagandha prior to this stress, the loss of neurons is reduced by 80 percent. You may recall that the hippocampus is critical for learning and memory, and the dense deposition of amyloid plaques and loss of neurons in the hippocampus that are seen in Alzheimer's dementia are thought to be major contributors to the profound disturbances of memory in the sufferers of this illness. In behavioral studies of rats designed as "preclinical" tests of new medications, ashwagandha was found to have effects similar to lorazepam, a medication prescribed for anxiety, and imipramine, an old and effective antidepressant medication. In diabetic rats, ashwagandha improves sensitivity to insulin, and it lowers cholesterol levels in rats made hypercholesterolemic by dietary methods. Thus, ashwagandha might be helpful in treating metabolic syndrome, which puts people at risk for dementia.

There are a handful of studies that show that ashwagandha can improve the cognitive function of laboratory animals, even when they suffer lesions similar to those seen in the brains of people with Alzheimer's dementia. Ashwagandha improved learning in mice, even after they were treated with a drug called scopolamine, which can produce dementia-like effects. While drugs prescribed to treat dementia increase acetylcholine activity, scopolamine blocks activity of certain acetylcholine receptors in the brain. Treatment with ashwagandha also improved memory in mice that had suffered damage after having had amyloid protein implanted in their brains.

Although it has been used to treat and prevent dementia in human patients, I note with some dismay that several companies that sell vitamins, herbs, and nutraceuticals have presented ashwagandha as if it were a tried and true remedy for dementia. They note its long use in Ayurvedic medicine and refer to results from animal studies as if they were human studies. Unfortunately, there are no reliable scientific studies showing that this extremely promising substance actually helps prevent or treat dementia in human beings.

Ashwagandha has been used since ancient times, and several reports have shown it to be safe in moderate doses. Thus, I doubt that there is any danger in trying it. Nonetheless, at this time I cannot recommend it. I am very much looking forward to seeing results from well-designed clinical studies.

CARNOSINE

Carnosine is a natural substance produced in the body and obtained in the diet of anyone who eats meat. Its primary usefulness is helping to prevent damage caused by too much sugar in the body. Sugars, such as glucose or fructose, can bind with proteins in a process called glycation. Glycation not only damages the protein, but also leads to proteins sticking to each other, or cross-linking. The destructive effects of protein glycation and cross-linking play major roles in the aging process. For example, cataracts, which tend to form in the lenses of the eyes as we age, are thought to be due to cross-linking of glycated proteins. This is the reason that cataracts are so common among sufferers of diabetes. Glycation and cross-linking also con-tribute to neurodegeneration and dementia.

Carnosine is formed in the body from the binding together of two amino acids, alanine and histidine. This pair of amino acids presents a binding site for glucose and other sugars that is very similar to sites where sugars tend to bind on complete proteins. Thus, carnosine can bind and contain sug-ars that might otherwise damage protein. The results of protein glycation, AGEs, go on to trigger inflammatory processes that in turn cause additional forms of cell damage. There is evidence that AGEs may also accelerate the production and accumulation of both beta amyloid and neurofibrillary tangles of tau protein. Deposits of those abnormal proteins in the brains of patients with Alzheimer's dementia almost invariably contain AGEs inter-mingled with the amyloid and tau.

Carnosine also has excellent antioxidant properties. It can greatly reduce damage from the highly reactive oxygen free radicals that are produced from the out-of-control oxidation of fats and sugars that can occur in meta-bolic syndrome and diabetes and which accelerate neurodegeneration in the brain. Carnosine also protects brain cells from triggering suicidal pro-grams of apoptosis under states of low oxygen as might occur in cardiovas-cular disease and vascular dementia. There is evidence from animal studies that carnosine can reduce the toxic effects of beta amyloid protein. Carno-sine has also been found to stimulate the activity of the enzyme carbonic anhydrase in the brain. This is an effect that is known to improve learning and memory in animals.

Brain tissue tends to have relatively high concentrations of carnosine. It has been suggested that the brain may be in particular need of the antigly-cation and antioxidant effects that carnosine provides. Interestingly, in nor-mal brains, carnosine levels are relatively high in the olfactory lobes. Those areas of the brain are often among the first to show damage in Alzheimer's dementia. I am not aware of studies of effects of carnosine in humans with Alzheimer's dementia. However, it is known that patients with Alzheimer's have blood levels of carnosine lower than those of healthy people of the same age.

Buying carnosine supplements may be an unnecessary inconvenience and expense when a person can obtain an adequate amount of carnosine simply by having meat once or twice a day. On the other hand, it has been found that strict vegetarians, who do not consume much carnosine in their diet, tend to have higher levels of glycosylated proteins in their bodies than do people who eat meat. Moreover, in people with diabetes, carnosine levels are lower than in people without diabetes, perhaps because it gets used up in its role of binding to excess glucose in the blood. Thus, vegetarians and people who suffer diabetes are particularly likely to benefit from carnosine supplementation. Some authors recommend taking 1000 mg of carnosine a day as a supplement. For comparison, a pound of beef contains about 1500 mg of carnosine. As a final word, I wish to note that most fish, such as salmon, are low in carnosine, but high in a substance called anserine. Anserine is also found in the human body and has actions in cells quite similar to those of carnosine.

CHOCOLATE

Chocolate had been cultivated by the Indians of Central America for thousands of years. It was the drink of the Indian aristocracy, and after it was brought back to Europe by the Spaniards, it became a drink of the European elite. In 1753, the Swedish taxonomist Linnaeus gave the cocoa plant the scientific name *Theobroma cacao*, which means "food of the gods." It remained expensive and difficult to obtain until the 1800s, when world trade and new processing methods made it more accessible for the common people.

Chocolate is rich in flavonoids. In fact it has more flavonoids than most foods, including tea or red wine. Flavonoids are molecules that are found in a variety of plants. The complex molecular structures of the flavonoids give them two important qualities. First, the multi-ringed flavonoid molecules absorb light in unique fashion and lend fruits and vegetables their deep, rich colors. Second, and more importantly, their molecular structure tends to make them powerful antioxidants. The flavonoids in chocolate are particularly potent antioxidants. Oxidation damages tissues, and it is largely responsible for the loss of function on the cellular level that leads to inflammation, protein damage, insulin resistance, mitochondrial damage, poor cellular function, and, eventually, cell death.

Flavonoids can interact with cellular chemistry in other important ways to help maintain health. Some benefits of chocolate flavonoids may come from their effects on a class of substances in the body known as eicosanoids. While all of the eicosanoids are important and necessary components of the body's arsenal for self defense, chronic overactivity of certain eicosanoids can lead to problems. Aspirin, ibuprofen, and other non-steroidal anti-inflammatory drugs (NSAIDs) produce their beneficial effects primarily by preventing the body from synthesizing eicosanoids that participate in inflammatory processes in the body. Flavonoids in chocolate tend to inhibit synthesis of a type of eicosanoid called leukotrienes. Leukotrienes act to constrict blood vessels, promote inflammation, and activate platelets. Overactive platelets predispose people to blood clots, heart attacks, and strokes. On the other hand, chocolate's flavonoids enhance synthesis of yet another class of eicosanoids, prostacyclins, which tend to enhance blood flow, prevent inflammation, and calm platelet activity. Regularly eating dark chocolate can reduce cardiac risk by nearly 20 percent through its ability to decrease LDL cholesterol oxidation, increase HDL cholesterol, reduce inflammation, decrease blood pressure, and dampen platelet activity. It also reduces insulin resistance. A recent study using magnetic resonance imaging showed that even in young, healthy women, drinking cocoa rich in flavonoids increased blood flow to the brain when the women were engaged in complex, cognitive tasks. By eating chocolate, one can help reduce the risk of metabolic syndrome, heart disease, and diabetes, and in turn reduce the risk of developing Alzheimer's, vascular, and other types of dementia.

Of particular interest are recent reports suggesting that chocolate may offer even more direct help in reducing the risk of dementia. Two of the major flavonoids in chocolate, epicatechin and catechin, have each been found to protect neurons from the toxic effects of exposure to the amyloid that accumulates in Alzheimer's dementia. Test tube studies have found that while each of these flavonoids alone offered neurons protection, when given together they enhanced each other's protective effects. Another test tube study published in 2008 found that epicatechin in chocolate inhibits activation of two chemical messengers of doom in brain cells, p38 MAPK and JNK. Apoptosis, the program of cellular suicide, is triggered in part by p38 MAPK and JNK. When epicatechin was added to the test tube, the activations of p38 MAPK and JNK in brain cells were prevented, and the apoptosis program of cell death was stopped.

I recommend eating a small piece of high quality, sugarless dark chocolate each day. Concern about the fat content of prepared chocolate is largely unwarranted. The cocoa butter mixed into chocolate to form bars contains a significant percentage of oleic acid, which is the healthy, monounsaturated fatty acid in olive oil. Although cocoa butter is rich in saturated fatty acids, about a third of that is the relatively benign saturated fat stearic acid. Stearic acid tends not to increase LDL cholesterol or decrease HDL cholesterol. In fact, the body is able to transform a significant portion of stearic acid directly into oleic acid. It has been found that the daily consumption of as much as 10 oz. of milk chocolate does not adversely affect serum cholesterol profiles. About 25 percent of the fat in cocoa butter is palmitic acid. Although palmitic acid is a natural product of our metabolism, it has few redeeming features. Nonetheless, any ill effects of the small amount of palmitic acid consumed in eating a piece of dark chocolate is counterbalanced by all of the beneficial effects of this remarkable food.

CHROMIUM

I must begin this section by informing you that there have been no studies of effects of chromium on Alzheimer's or other types of dementia, nor is there any direct evidence that chromium can be used to prevent or treat dementia of any kind. A study performed in Italy showed that adequate levels of chromium, among other trace minerals, correlated with maintenance of cognitive function in the elderly. However, there was no clear indication to what degree chromium itself may have contributed to that effect. With that being said, I will tell you my belief that chromium supplementation has been overlooked as an easy, natural, and inexpensive way to help prevent metabolic syndrome and diabetes type 2, which are major risk factors for dementia. There is also published evidence that chromium can help relieve certain forms of depression, which, in turn, can decrease the risk of dementia. Because supplementation of the diet with chromium may help reduce the likelihood of several major risk factors for dementia, it stands to reason that it may help prevent dementia as well.

In 1959, Dr. Walter Mertz proposed that chromium is an essential trace mineral and that it plays a role in enhancing the activity of insulin. People lacking in chromium have high serum glucose levels that require high levels of insulin to bring glucose levels under control. That is, they are resistant to insulin, which is the underlying characteristic of metabolic syndrome.

When chromium levels are normalized, high glucose levels are reduced and sensitivity to insulin is restored. Chromium, usually in the form of chromium picolinate in doses of 200 to 1000 micrograms a day, is sufficient to improve glucose tolerance. Chromium also lowers serum triglycerides and increases good (HDL) cholesterol in patients with diabetes type 2.

Chromium has been successfully used to treat both major depression and dysthymia, which is a mild but persistent form of depression. The type of depression that is most responsive to treatment with chromium is often referred to as atypical depression. This is a form of depression that is more common in women than men, and it is characterized by depressed mood, lack of motivation, low sex drive, sleeping too much, carbohydrate craving, and weight gain. Along with improvement in mood, the strongest effects of chromium in such patients are countering the three symptoms of carbohydrate craving, high appetite, and low sex drive. There is some evidence that chromium might produce these benefits by affecting certain subtypes of receptors responsive to the neurotransmitter serotonin. However, I and other researchers suspect that these benefits are primarily due to increases in the sensitivity of insulin receptors in the brain.

It is thought that most people consume sufficient amounts of chromium. However, certain circumstances can cause people to not utilize chromium properly. Too much iron in the body may prevent transport and effective use of chromium. There is also evidence that the elderly may not utilize chromium efficiently. Of particular interest are animal studies showing that under conditions of hyperglycemia and increased demand for insulin, such as occur in metabolic syndrome, there is an increase in loss of chromium in the urine. Thus, a lack of sufficient chromium may contribute to metabolic syndrome, which in turn increases loss of chromium and further exacerbates metabolic syndrome in a vicious cycle.

A number of years ago there were some troubling reports that chromium picolinate can cause chromosomal damage in an animal model. This effect did not seem to be due to chromium itself, as other forms of chromium, for example, chromium nicotinate, did not do this. It is important to state that several subsequent studies have found that the common dose of 400 micrograms of chromium picolinate daily for eight weeks has no damaging effects on the DNA. In my psychiatric practice I quite often advise patients to take 200 micrograms of chromium a day, especially when depressed mood is accompanied by evidence of metabolic syndrome. I am hopeful that research will be done to see if this inexpensive and well-tolerated mineral does indeed reduce the risk of dementia.

CO-ENZYME Q10

Co-enzyme Q10 (CoQ10) is natural to the body and essential for life. It is a molecule that forms part of what is known as the electron transport chain in the mitochondria of every cell in the body. It is essential for the production of energy. The basic chemistry of oxidation itself involves the transfer of electrons. Thus, because of CoQ10's role in the electron transport chain, it is also perfectly suited as an antioxidant.

Blood levels of CoQ10 do not appear to change either with age or with changes in cognitive function. Blood levels are the same in patients with Alzheimer's as in normal, age-matched control subjects. However, levels of the substance have been found to decrease in brain tissue as people age. There are a number of animal studies showing that supplementation with CoQ10 can have neuroprotective effects on the brain.

One might expect that, due to CoQ10's role as an energy-producing molecule in the mitochondria, the neuroprotective effects would arise primarily from CoQ10-induced increases in energy production in the mitochondria. In one study, treating old, diabetic rats with CoQ10 helped increase the energy production of their mitochondria. However, the benefits of CoQ10 supplementation are more clearly the result of antioxidant and other effects of this substance. Adding CoQ10 to the diets of old mice greatly reduced the presence of substances known to be the result of oxidative damage in their brains. In old mice genetically engineered to express abnormal proteins similar to those in humans with Alzheimer's dementia, CoQ10 helped protect brain tissue from oxidative damage due to loss of blood supply. In test tube studies, CoQ10 helped to dissolve fibers of amyloid protein that had formed in rat brain tissue. It also helps prevent the toxic effects of amyloid deposits in brain tissue. Studies on the effects of CoQ10 on learning and memory in living animals are sparse. However, one study showed that while neither CoQ10 nor vitamin E alone were beneficial, combined treatment significantly improved learning and memory in old mice.

CoQ10 supplementation has been reported to reduce oxidative stress and chemical markers of inflammation in animal models of the metabolic syndrome. This is less clear in human subjects. However, a study has shown that giving people already diagnosed with metabolic syndrome 60 mg of CoQ10 for eight weeks significantly reduced their fasting insulin levels, blood sugar, triglycerides, and evidence of oxidative damage.

Most studies of the use of CoQ10 in human neurodegenerative diseases have been in patients with Parkinson's disease, Huntington's disease, and the rare neurological disorder called Friedreich's ataxia. Some promising effects of CoQ10 supplementation have been reported for each of these illnesses. However, while these illnesses can have cognitive and psychiatric components, they are not generally thought of as forms of dementia. To the best of my knowledge, there have not been formal studies of the effects of CoQ10 supplementation on Alzheimer's, vascular, Lewy body, or fronto-temporal forms of dementia.

Studies have shown that CoQ10 is safe and well tolerated, and supplementing with 200 to 400 mg a day is typical. I wish to note that the synthesis of CoQ10 and cholesterol by the body share similar steps and enzymatic pathways. For that reason, the statin class of medications used to lower blood levels of cholesterol by blocking its synthesis also tend to decrease body levels of CoQ10. Thus, people taking a statin to control their cholesterol should ask their doctors about supplementing with several hundred milligrams a day of CoQ10 to prevent depletion of this critical substance. I must note that in individuals with chronically low levels of oxygen in their brains due to congestive heart disease, chronic obstructive pulmonary disease, severe sleep apnea, vascular dementia, or other causes, it might be better to supplement with idebenone instead of CoQ10. Idebenone is discussed later in this chapter.

COFFEE

I am happy to inform you that there are several studies showing that people who drink two to four cups of coffee each day are less likely to develop Alzheimer's dementia than are people who do not drink coffee. Exactly how coffee might help to prevent or delay Alzheimer's dementia is unclear. However, scientific studies have shown that caffeine and other substances in coffee have a number of different effects on the brain that would be expected to improve one's chances of avoiding dementia. For example, there is evidence that caffeine can reduce the burden and detrimental effects of beta amyloid on the brain. APPsw Swedish mutation mice have been genetically engineered to develop many of the same plaques and tangles in their brains that are seen in humans with Alzheimer's dementia. These mice also exhibit premature losses in memory and learning functions, in ways very similar to those that occur in Alzheimer's patients. The addition of caffeine to their drinking water, in amounts equivalent to five cups of coffee a day, both decreased the amount of beta amyloid that accumulated in their brains and prevented decline in cognitive function. In a similar type of study, treatment with caffeine blocked the loss of cognitive functions caused by microinjections of beta amyloid protein into the brains of otherwise normal mice.

Coffee reduces inflammation and improves the health of the endothelial lining of arteries. Some substances in coffee also have significant antioxidant effects. Together, these beneficial effects of coffee offer the brain protection from some of the primary pathological processes that cause Alzheimer's and other neurodegenerative diseases to progress. These effects would also tend to help prevent metabolic syndrome, heart disease, diabetes, and other conditions that increase the risk of dementia. For the sake of completeness, I must note that some studies have shown that coffee can increase serum cholesterol. This is particularly the case when the coffee is made by methods that don't use paper filters, such as the French press method. Although reports are inconsistent, there are also studies suggesting that drinking coffee can decrease insulin sensitivity, which would increase the risk of metabolic syndrome. Nonetheless, a recent study in France found that drinking coffee can reduce the risk of developing diabetes type 2 by nearly a half. Perhaps the best advice would be to drink coffee that has been brewed with the use of unbleached paper filters, which is the type of coffee least likely to adversely affect cholesterol.

For me, the primary concern about drinking coffee is that consuming caffeine too late in the day can interfere with sleep. I recommend against drinking caffeinated beverages after six o'clock in the evening. Some people can experience mild agitation or even heart palpitations if they drink too much coffee. If this happens to you, decrease it or stop drinking it. Finally, I wish to note that I have feverishly been poring through the scientific literature hoping to find some indication that half-and-half might also be of some benefit to sufferers or potential sufferers of dementia. Unfortunately, I have found no evidence that this is the case.

CURCUMIN

Curcumin, a component of the spice turmeric, has recently been touted in the lay literature to be a substance of great promise in the treatment of inflammatory illnesses, diabetes, and metabolic syndrome. A natural substance acting in a multitude of beneficial ways without obvious ill effects is a very appealing possibility.

Evidence in the literature consists primarily of animal studies. However, the curcumin data looks quite encouraging. For example, in diabetic rats, curcumin reversed many of the liver dysfunctions that lead to hyperglycemia. Curcumin also lowers cholesterol and triglycerides in diabetic rats. Of substantial interest is the report, again from rat studies, that curcumin stimulates PPAR-gamma, the activity of which is thought to greatly benefit sufferers of metabolic syndrome and diabetes type 2.

Curcumin has anticancer and antioxidant effects, as well as anti-inflammatory properties, due to its ability to block the activities of NF-κB, cyclooxygenase, and nitric oxide synthase. Cyclooxygenase inhibitors have usefulness in the treatment of arthritic conditions. It is of interest to note that most prescribed antidepressants have the ability to block nitric oxide synthase activity in the brain, and some authors suspect that this effect is at least partially responsible for their ability to improve mood.

New evidence shows that curcumin may also have usefulness in the treatment of Alzheimer's disease. In the test tube, curcumin appears to break up the aggregations of amyloid fibers. Most impressively, when it is injected into aged rats with Alzheimer's-like plaques of amyloid, those plaques begin to reduce in size. In a study from Singapore, where the people often consume curry dishes rich in the spice turmeric, it has been found that elderly people who regularly consume curry dishes perform better on the MMSE test of cognitive function than do those who do not indulge in this flavorful dish.

The first formal study of the effects of curcumin on cognitive function in human subjects diagnosed with mild Alzheimer's dementia, however, has been disappointing. This study, performed by Dr. John Ringman in the UCLA laboratory of Dr. Jeffrey Cummings, found no significant ability of curcumin to improve or slow down the loss of cognitive function in those subjects. Ringman informed me that the low bioavailability of curcumin, that is, the relatively small amount of the substance that was actually absorbed into the bloodstream of subjects, may have limited any beneficial effects. In any case, research will continue.

Thankfully, safety concerns have been addressed at this point in time, and existing evidence indicates that curcumin is fairly safe in humans. There have been reports that high doses can cause stomach ulcers in rats. Thus, it would seem prudent for people with a history of gastric ulcers to avoid curcumin. In most cases, however, even enormous doses of curcumin fed to laboratory rats have been found to do little more than turn their fur yellow. As noted by Ringman, the most difficult limiting factor in the use of curcumin may be that it is very poorly absorbed. Hopefully, a way will be found for oral dosing to provide therapeutic blood levels of the substance.

CYTIDINE 5'-DIPHOSPHOCHOLINE (CDP-CHOLINE)

In dementia, particularly the Alzheimer's and Lewy body forms of the illness, loss of cognitive function is thought to be due in part to decreases in brain levels of the neurotransmitter acetylcholine. There are two ways to increase levels of acetylcholine in the brain. One way is to prevent the destruction of the neurotransmitter by blocking the activity of the cholinesterase enzymes. Most of the drugs that are FDA approved for the treatment of dementia act to increase acetylcholine in this manner. Another way to increase acetylcholine is to increase the amount of the neurotransmitter that is made in the brain. Cytidine 5'-diphosphocholine (CDP-choline) is one of several compounds that increase tissue levels of choline, which the brain uses to make acetylcholine.

CDP-choline is formed naturally in the body. Along with supplying choline to produce acetylcholine, CDP-choline also provides the material to produce phosphatidylcholine in the brain. Phosphatidylcholine is a critical component in cell membranes. It is thought that when the brain is running low on acetylcholine, phosphatidylcholine in cell membranes is cannibalized to make more of the needed neurotransmitter. In some cases, the cell membrane may be so compromised by loss of phosphatidylcholine that the cell loses function and dies. Whereas some of the effect of CDP-choline is to replenish acetylcholine, many scientists suspect that the more important role of CDP-choline is preventing depletion of phosphatidylcholine, which is necessary to maintain the integrity of the cell membrane. In studies using laboratory rats, treatment with CDP-choline has been found to significantly increase not only brain levels of phosphatidylcholine, but also those of the related substances phosphatidylserine and phosphatidylethanolamine. As I describe in a section below, treatment with phosphatidylserine itself is known to improve cognitive function in people suffering dementia.

Treatment with CPD-choline appears to have a protective effect against the damage that amyloid protein can cause in the brain. In rats that received microinjections of amyloid into their hippocampus, pretreatment with CPD-choline prevented the inflammation and cell death that was seen in the brains of untreated rats. Treatment with CPD-choline also appears to help prevent the buildup of amyloid protein as is seen in the plaques that accumulate in the brains of patients with Alzheimer's dementia. Normal phosphatidylcholine concentrations in the cell membrane are thought to be necessary for the cell to secrete amyloid in forms that can be carried out of the brain rather than being left to build up and form plaques.

It is known that the brain is particularly vulnerable to destruction of phosphatidylcholine in cell membranes of neurons during periods of hypoxia that occur in strokes. The Cochrane reviewers reviewed existing reports on the effects of CDP-choline and found that it can help improve cognitive function in patients with mild to moderate vascular dementia. It is somewhat disappointing that CDP-choline has not been shown to offer much benefit to sufferers of Alzheimer's dementia. Some improvements may be noticeable, but no statistically significant differences have been seen between those who receive CDP-choline and those who do not. I have not seen studies in which CDP-choline has been added to standard medical treatments of Alzheimer's dementia, such as administration of cholinesterase inhibitors or memantine. There is no obvious reason why CDP-choline could not be added to those treatments, and there is reason to suspect that it could enhance the effects of those medications. Because CDP-choline would increase the availability of choline to produce acetylcholine, it might be particularly effective in enhancing the effects of the cholinesterase inhibitors. On a more optimistic note, several well-controlled studies have shown that a month or two of supplementation with CDP-choline can improve memory function in elderly individuals with mild cognitive impairment. It is not known if benefits include preventing or delaying progression of MCI into actual dementia.

CDP-choline is available in health food stores and on the Internet. The dose of CDP-choline that has generally been used and found to be effective in improving cognitive function in scientific studies is 1000 mg a day. I have seen no reports that this dose has any adverse effects. In view of the fact that this substance is natural and produced in the body, it is likely that moderate doses of CDP-choline are entirely safe.

DHEA

DHEA stands for dehydroepiandrosterone. Like the stress hormone cortisol, DHEA is a steroid synthesized in the adrenal glands. It has been found to counteract some of the adverse effects of cortisol, and it may be one of the body's methods to control the stress response. DHEA can also be converted into other steroid hormones, including ones with actions similar to the sex hormones estrogen and testosterone. Estrogen and testosterone are themselves steroid hormones, though they are produced in the ovaries and testes rather than the adrenal glands.

Blood levels of DHEA peak around the age of twenty and drop rapidly after the age of twenty-five. A rather sobering finding has been that abnormally low levels of DHEA correlate with an increased risk of dying within the subsequent five to ten years. Some studies have disputed that finding, however, and no studies have shown that restoring normal DHEA levels in any way extends life span in such individuals. Nonetheless, DHEA has acquired a reputation for improving a variety of human inadequacies, from depression to sexual dysfunction to poor cognitive function to loss of youthful vitality. Its use is growing in the United States, and it is often available over the counter in the neighborhood drug or grocery store. I suspect that if it were only now being made available, it would be by prescription only.

There are a number of properties of DHEA that have generated interest in its potential to prevent and treat dementia. DHEA blocks neurotoxic effects of amyloid in rat brain. It also stimulates the brain to produce healthier forms of amyloid that are less likely to stick and form plaques. When the body lacks sufficient DHEA, the accumulation of toxic beta amyloid accelerates. It has been found to stimulate the birth of neurons by neurogenesis in rat brain and, at the same time, to protect neurons from self-programmed death by apoptosis. A single study shows similar neural-growth-stimulating effects of DHEA in human brain cells. There is evidence that a metabolite of DHEA, dehydroepiandrosterone sulfate, enhances the activity of the neurotransmitter acetylcholine, which is deficient in most forms of dementia. DHEA also enhances long-term potentiation, which is the biochemical process that underlies learning in the mammalian brain.

There are studies showing that DHEA can improve learning and memory in aging animals and in those genetically engineered to suffer deficits similar to those seen in Alzheimer's dementia. DHEA improves learning and memory in SAMP8 mice, which are seen as an animal model of Alzheimer's dementia. In another study, DHEA improved cognitive function in old rats, but not in young healthy rats. DHEA has even been found to improve memory in day-old chicks.

Studies of the relationships between blood levels of DHEA and cognitive abilities have been rather inconsistent. However, by and large, they have tended to show a relationship between low DHEA and increased likelihood of diminished cognitive function and dementia. In one study, it was found that across a wide range of ages, women with higher blood levels of DHEA scored better in tests of cognitive function than did women with lower levels of the hormone. In a study of men, subjects who were diagnosed as having Alzheimer's dementia had significantly lower levels of DHEA than did men who did not suffer the illness. In a study with contrary findings, no such relationships between blood levels of DHEA and level of cognitive function were seen in men over the age of seventy-five who had already been diagnosed with Alzheimer's dementia. It is worth noting that in yet another study, DHEA levels were no different in men with or without dementia, but ratios of DHEA to the stress hormone cortisol were significantly lower in men with Alzheimer's dementia. That study suggested that DHEA levels can be normal, yet too low to counteract adverse effects of cortisol in certain individuals suffering stress. One of the more interesting studies involved measurement of DHEA levels not in blood, but in brain tissue itself. In that study, it was found that DHEA and its metabolites were reduced in concentration in various areas of the brain and that low levels of the hormone correlated with higher concentrations of amyloid plaque and neurofibrillary tangles of tau protein in those areas.

From much of the data described above it might be concluded that DHEA would be a perfect treatment to help prevent and improve dementia. Unfortunately, as was so aptly noted by the great English biologist Thomas Huxley, "Many a beautiful theory has been destroyed by an ugly fact." The ugly fact in this case is that, in actuality, supplementing with DHEA neither prevents nor improves dementia. The much anticipated DHEA and Wellness (DAWN) Trial concluded with the impression that "DHEA supplementation has no benefit on cognitive performance or well-being in healthy older adults, and it should not be recommended for that purpose in the general population." The Cochrane reviewers conveyed a similar understanding in stating, "The data offer no support at present for an improvement in memory or other aspects of cognitive function following DHEA treatment in normal older people." In one study of post-menopausal women, DHEA was even suspected of worsening cognitive function.

There is evidence that DHEA can help major depression in some individuals. There is also evidence that DHEA can increase testosterone levels and thus increase sex drive, particularly in women. As a psychiatrist, I have several times recommended DHEA for those purposes. There is also some evidence that DHEA can improve certain aspects of metabolic syndrome, which may be due in part to a natural antagonist effect toward cortisol. DHEA may improve insulin sensitivity and reduce inflammation. It may also help reduce the burden of visceral fat. All in all, however, I can not recommend it for use in preventing or treating dementia. The scientific support isn't there.

FISH OIL (OMEGA-3 FATTY ACIDS, EPA, DHA)

The human body stores energy for future use in two different ways. One way is to link sugar molecules together to form the animal starch molecule called glycogen. This process takes place primarily in the liver and, to far lesser extent, in muscle cells. Glycogen has the advantage of being able to very quickly be broken down into glucose for use as energy. However, glycogen is not a very efficient way to store calories. Ounce for ounce, far more energy can be stored in fat than in glycogen, and through millions of years of evolution, the production and deposition of fat has become the primary means to pack away unused calories.

The body can readily convert unused carbohydrate into fatty acids, which are long chains of carbon and hydrogen with an oxygen-containing acid group on the end.[1] The acid group makes the end soluble in the watery environment of the cell, which in turn helps to position the fatty acid in proper place, as well as to provide a chemical "handle" to carry the fatty acid into various chemical reactions in the cell. Under normal circumstances, there are only two basic types of fatty acids in the body. In one type, each carbon in the chain binds to a maximal number of hydrogen atoms, and is thus "saturated" with hydrogen. In the other type, some carbons share extra chemical bonds with each other rather than to the maximal number of hydrogens, and they are referred to as "unsaturated" fatty acids. When only two carbons share an extra bond, the fatty acid is monounsaturated; when this occurs two or more times in a molecule, the fatty acid is described as polyunsaturated. The differences in energy content between saturated and unsaturated acids are trivial. However, these types of fatty acids are quite different from each other in their chemistries and in the ways in which the body can put them to use when not simply using them for fuel.

The main product of the conversion of carbohydrate to fat is the saturated fatty acid palmitate. The body can also produce monounsaturated fatty acids from saturated fats that it either synthesizes or obtains in food. Among the most noteworthy monounsaturated fats the body can produce in this way is oleic acid, which is one of the fatty acids in olive oil.

There are two types of fatty acids that the body cannot synthesize, the polyunsaturated omega-3 and omega-6 fatty acids.[2] These are the so-called essential fatty acids, and we must obtain them from our diet to maintain good health. The only truly essential omega-3 fatty acid is alpha-linolenic

---

1. Petroleum and refined petroleum products, such as gasoline and kerosene, are also mixtures of chains of carbon and hydrogen, or what are commonly referred to as hydrocarbons. Although the "burning" of hydrocarbons in the body is slower and far more controlled than what occurs in a spontaneous combustion engine, the fundamental molecular source of energy is the same.

2. The Greek letter *omega* is the name given to the end carbon in a fatty acid chain, and the number, such as omega-3 or omega-6, refers to where the extra carbon-carbon bond in an unsaturated fatty acid lies in relation to the omega carbon.

acid, which is found in seed oils, such as from flax. The human body is able to use alpha-linolenic acid to make other omega-3 fatty acids it needs. Omega-6 fatty acids are also found in seed and grain oils, such as from corn, canola, and safflower. The only essential omega-6 fatty acid is arachidonic acid, from which the body makes other necessary omega-6 fatty acids.

While both omega-3 and omega-6 fatty acids are essential, they are different from one another. Both are necessary to produce a number of critical chemical messengers in the body. The powerful hormone-like substances called eicosanoids are produced from both omega-3 and omega-6 fatty acids. However, the eicosanoids derived from omega-6 fatty acids tend to have inflammatory effects, whereas those derived from omega-3 fatty acids tend to dampen inflammation. An over-abundance of omega-6 relative to omega-3 fatty acids puts us at risk for inflammatory states. Thus, we are faced not only with providing ourselves adequate amounts of the essential fatty acids, but also obtaining them in proper proportion. Unfortunately, the ratio of omega-3 to omega-6 polyunsaturated fatty acids in our diet has changed through the centuries. The polyunsaturated fats from the vegetable oils we commonly consume from salads and cooked foods are unbalanced in terms of containing too much omega-6.

The body can use alpha-linolenic acid to produce two other extremely important omega-3 fatty acids, eicosapentaenoic acid (EPA) and docosahexaenoic acid (DHA). It is EPA and DHA that are found in deep-sea fish oil. However, while the body is capable of turning alpha-linolenic acid into EPA and DHA, it is not terribly efficient in doing so. It is for this reason that including fish in the diet, or simply supplementing the diet with fish oil capsules, is so important.

A wealth of studies shows that optimizing intake of the omega-3 fatty acids EPA and DHA can improve various aspects of metabolic syndrome. EPA and DHA help relieve hypertension and maintain insulin sensitivity in normal subjects. Fish oil is well known to reduce serum triglycerides and increase good HDL cholesterol. Omega-3 fatty acids also help reduce many of the secondary effects of metabolic syndrome, such as inflammation. Blood markers of inflammation, including C-reactive protein (CRP) and TNF-alpha, are lowered by fish oil. This may be the result of enhanced synthesis of anti-inflammatory prostaglandins. Inflammation is a risk factor for dementia, as is metabolic syndrome.

Omega-3 fatty acids protect the brain from degeneration. They decrease oxidative stress and dampen inflammation. In rats, DHA is able to disrupt deposits of amyloid in brain tissue and to decrease levels of amyloid. EPA stimulates production of some of the enzymes involved in neurogenesis.

On the other hand, brain cells in rats fed diets supplemented with EPA are better able to withstand stress and hypoxia, and thereby resist apoptosis triggered by partial loss of blood supply.

Saturated animal fat in the diet increases the risk of developing Alzheimer's disease. Consumption of fish containing high levels of omega-3 fatty acid counteracts some of that risk. People who consume fish at least once a week can have a 60 percent reduction in the likelihood of developing Alzheimer's disease. Curiously, this protective effect of fish consumption is not seen in individuals who carry the APOE4 gene, which is known to predispose carriers to Alzheimer's disease. It is not clear why this is the case.

The fact that blood levels of DHA and EPA are often lower in Alzheimer's patients than in normal subjects further suggests that these fatty acids might be useful in treating Alzheimer's dementia. Unfortunately, treatment of Alzheimer's patients with fish oil or other omega-3 fatty acid preparations, such as ethyl-EPA, have been disappointing. It is possible that by the time the illness is diagnosed, the damage is already done. I suspect that fish oil is more useful in preventing rather than treating dementia.

Given the fact that fish oil has been part of the human diet for thousands of generations, I believe it can be said that consuming deep-sea fish and supplementing with fish oil capsules is perfectly safe. I must note that along with raising good HDL cholesterol, fish oil also slightly increases LDL cholesterol, which has led some physicians to cast a wary eye upon its use. However, while increasing levels of total LDL, it also tends to increase the size of LDL particles, which makes them less harmful. There may also be legitimate concerns about ingesting unsafe levels of mercury or other heavy metals in a diet that includes frequent meals of fish. The content of mercury varies among species of ocean fish. As a rule of thumb, it is the large predatory fish high in ocean food chain, such as tuna, swordfish, marlin, and shark, that are most susceptible to accumulating heavy metals in their flesh. Many species of fish, including salmon, herring, flounder, cod, and sardines, present little danger from heavy metals. Well-known brands of fish oil capsules are generally free of such contaminants. Overall, the benefits of consuming fish or supplementing with fish oil capsules far outweigh the risks. I generally instruct my patients to supplement their diet with 3 grams a day of a good brand of deep-sea fish oil.

GARLIC

It is said that a meal without garlic is a like a bell without a clapper. How fortunate that garlic is not only magnificent on the palate, but also so good for us. The origin of human use of garlic to flavor our food has been lost in antiquity. However, the use of garlic is mentioned in the Old Testament and in the ancient writings of the Egyptians, Greeks, and Romans. I personally suspect that Neanderthal pioneers of haute cuisine chopped up wild garlic to flavor their mastodon burgers.

M. Grieve's wonderful *A Modern Herbal*, first published in 1931, describes a wide variety of medicinal uses of garlic throughout human history. She describes among its attributes antiseptic, stimulant, diaphoretic, and diuretic effects. She also recalls the Homeric legend that having consumed some garlic saved Ulysses from being transformed into a pig by the sorceress Circe. This would seem to be protection of which we would all be wise to take advantage. Although some critical human data is lacking, there are more scientifically valid reasons to believe that garlic can help reduce the risk of Alzheimer's, vascular, and other forms of dementia.

Like its cousins onions and shallots, garlic contains a variety of sulfur-containing biochemicals that not only give it its pungent odor, but some remarkable medicinal properties as well. There is evidence, however, that the well-known and much maligned odor of garlic on the breath is not necessary to gain the benefits of garlic. Aging garlic appears to both reduce its odor and transform some of its constituent chemicals into others that may be even more effective in their antioxidant and anti-inflammatory effects. For example, with aging, the odiferous allicin in fresh garlic is converted into the somewhat more pleasant substances S-allylcysteine, diallyl-disulfide, and S-allylmercaptocysteine. Extracts of aged garlic are available in pharmacies, health food stores, and on the Internet. It is not clear that the benefits of aged garlic over fresh garlic are so great or unique to make their purchase and use the obvious choice over simply making an effort to use more of the far less expensive fresh garlic in your daily diet. Nonetheless, most of the studies on effects of garlic that might be relevant to preventing dementia have been performed with aged garlic.

Among the effects of garlic that might be expected to help prevent dementia are powerful antioxidant effects, as well as stimulation of enzymes, such as superoxide dismutase, catalase, and glutathione peroxidase, that offer natural antioxidant protection in the body. There is also evidence that some of the sulfur-bearing substances in garlic are readily converted into the brain-protective gas hydrogen sulfide in the brain and other tissues of the body. Garlic helps prevent oxidation of lipids and also appears to have significant anti-inflammatory effects. Aged garlic reduces blood pressure and increases blood flow, likely by improving health of the endothelial lining of blood vessels. Aged garlic has also been shown to lower bad LDL cholesterol and increase good HDL cholesterol. It may do this by blocking the activity of the enzyme HMG-CoA, which produces cholesterol. The statins prescribed to lower cholesterol also act by blocking this enzyme. However, it is thought that garlic may affect HMG-CoA in a different way than the statins do, and may thus be additive to them in the reduction of serum cholesterol.

I do note that not all studies of effects of garlic on cholesterol or blood pressure in men and women are positive. For example, one very recent study in the well regarded *Archives of Internal Medicine* found that neither raw garlic, up to four cloves a day for six months, nor aged garlic improved cholesterol levels in adults with mild hypercholesterolemia. A large "meta-analysis," that is, a study in which the results of many separate studies are combined and analyzed by sophisticated statistical methods, found garlic to have no beneficial effects on blood pressure. However, the authors of that study still believed that garlic held promise as a means to reduce heart disease.

Of particular significance are reports that extracts of aged garlic can prevent the death of cultured neuron-like cells that are exposed to beta amyloid protein. In mice genetically altered to develop a constellation of symptoms very similar to Alzheimer's dementia in humans, treatment with aged garlic extract reduces the amounts of both beta amyloid plaque and neurofibrillary tangles of hyperphosphorylated tau protein. In this same type of mouse, often referred to as the Alzheimer Tg2576 transgenic mouse, treatment with aged garlic also prevents the decreases in learning and memory functions that emerge in these animals as they age. Interestingly, at least one study found that giving aged garlic at an early stage in the progression of plaques and tangles in these transgenic mice, a stage that might be similar to the MCI stage in humans, was effective in preventing or at least delaying deficits in learning and memory. Unfortunately, there are no studies of how garlic, either raw or in the form of extracts of aged garlic, affect the progression of Alzheimer's or other forms of dementia in human subjects. However, the available scientific data is encouraging, and since garlic is delicious in food and reasonable amounts are perfectly safe, I would suggest that you use garlic at every opportunity to enhance the flavor of your food. I do not believe that there is yet sufficient evidence of the ability of garlic to prevent or delay dementia to warrant buying the more expensive extracts of aged garlic to take as a supplement.

GINKGO

The ginkgo tree, which biologists refer to by the scientific name *Ginkgo biloba*, is often referred to as a living fossil. It has descended largely unchanged from ancestors that lived over 250 million years ago. Its odd, fan-like leaves have a primitive, yet graceful appearance. Another interesting characteristic of the ginkgo tree is that the species is dioecious, that is, individual trees are either male or female. The ginkgo has been used for food as well as for medicinal purposes for thousands of years. One of the most frequently cited uses in Chinese medicine is for asthma and other respiratory disorders. There are alleged to also be ancient references to its use for improving memory; however, I have not found reliable sources to verify this. In the 1980s, an extract of *Ginkgo biloba* called EGb 761 became very popular in Germany as a treatment for memory loss. The mechanism of action was thought to be the ability of the herb to increase blood flow to the brain. In 1988 alone, German doctors wrote more than 5 million prescriptions for EGb 761. In the late 1980s, ginkgo also became a popular treatment for memory loss in the United States.

Extracts of *Ginkgo biloba* contain a variety of substances known as flavonoids and terpenoids, which appear to have medicinal properties. Test tube data has strongly suggested that ginkgo contains substances that could block or reverse several different neurodegenerative processes that lead to loss of cognitive function. One of the most well-documented effects of ginkgo is improvement in blood flow, probably due to its ability to relax smooth muscle cells in the lining of small arteries. It is believed that ginkgo can improve blood supply to the brain and improve cognitive function in individuals whose blood supply is compromised. This is not uncommon in elderly patients. Another well-known effect is a decrease in the likelihood of blood clotting, which is due to the terpene molecule ginkoglideB blocking some of the effects of platelet-activating factor (PAF). Platelets are cell-like structures in the blood that stick together and initiate clotting of blood. PAF also participates in triggering some inflammatory processes, and it is thought to play a role in some of the damaging effects of inflammation on neurons in the brains of patients with various forms of neurodegenerative dementia. Ginkgo has been found to reduce the inflammatory damage stimulated by amyloid deposition in brain tissue, which was thought to be due to its ability to block the effects of PAF. There are also a number of reports that ginkgo extracts can also slow the growth rate of amyloid deposits in the brain, though it is not known how this might occur. When amyloid begins to build up in brain tissue, it can prevent the release of acetylcholine, which is necessary for normal cognitive functioning. Ginkgo helps restore acetylcholine release in brain tissue exposed to amyloid. Although extract of ginkgo can inhibit acetylcholinesterase, which is the mechanism of action of most of the FDA-approved medications for dementia, it does so only at very high concentrations, thus I doubt that it acts in this way in people using the herb. Ginkgo is also an antioxidant and free radical scavenger, which would make a ginkgo extract an excellent defense against the damage of oxidative stress. There is also a report that ginkgo stimulates neurogenesis in the brains of mice that have been genetically altered to develop amyloid plaques in their brains very similar to those that develop in people with Alzheimer's dementia.

Treatment with *Ginkgo biloba* extract improves learning and memory in both young and old rats. It also improves learning and memory in rats that are stressed during the learning of their behavioral tasks. Perhaps most impressive are results showing that treatment with ginkgo can improve learning and memory in the mice that are studied as animal models of Alzheimer's dementia.

Together, the scientifically established effects of ginkgo on the brain and its blood supply, as well as results from animal studies of learning and memory, would suggest that it could offer significant benefits in the prevention and treatment of vascular and Alzheimer's dementia. Several studies have shown that ginkgo is helpful in the treatment of dementia. In one recent study performed in 2007, the ginkgo extract EGb 761 was found to improve cognitive function in patients with mild to moderate vascular or Alzheimer's dementia. Another study in 2007 found EGb 761 to have effects equal to those of the prescribed medication Aricept in slowing the rate of decline in patients with moderately severe Alzheimer's dementia.

Unfortunately, the clinical data has not been consistent in showing an ability to prevent cognitive loss in normal elderly subjects or to improve cognitive function in patients already diagnosed with Alzheimer's dementia. In 2007, the Cochrane reviewers stated that reported effects of ginkgo on dementia are "inconsistent and unconvincing." One of the most recent and disappointing studies, funded by the Alzheimer's Society and published in the June 2008 issue of the *International Journal of Geriatric Psychiatry*, found that six months of treatment with "a standard dose of high purity *Ginkgo biloba*" offered no benefits whatsoever in relieving or preventing progression of cognitive symptoms in patients with mild to moderate Alzheimer's dementia. Another recent study published in the *Journal of the American Medical Association* casts doubt on the usefulness of ginkgo in dementia. Over a period of five years, a group of over three thousand subjects over seventy-five years of age were given either ginkgo or placebo capsules and then monitored for changes in cognitive function. There was absolutely no difference between those groups in the number of people who later developed dementia.

Some of the good that ginkgo likely does by decreasing the activity of platelets also leads to the possibility of the herb causing problems in some people. The major concern is bleeding. Although not completely substantiated, ginkgo has been implicated in a number of cases in which individuals suffered significant bleeding events while taking the herb. There are a number of important studies still being conducted on potential benefits of ginkgo. However, because of potential danger due to bleeding, lack of clear evidence of its benefit, and availability of other supplements that do appear to be helpful without significant risks, I cannot at this time recommend using ginkgo to treat or prevent dementia.

GINSENG

Ginseng has been used as medicine in Asia for thousands of years. It has often been used as a restorative, tonic medicine for the elderly. The most commonly used forms are Asian ginseng and American ginseng. They are similar in their effects, although Asian ginseng is often said to be more potent than the American plant. As is often the case with herbal medicines, the extracts of ginseng are extremely complicated in makeup. They always contain a variety of related compounds, referred to as ginsenosides or saponins. The different extraction processes, sources, and types of ginseng can result in significant differences in the concentrations or even the very presence of important medicinal components of the ginseng. Standardized extracts from reputable herbal medicine sources should be used.

There are many studies showing that supplementation with ginseng can reduce the risk of metabolic syndrome, which in turn is one of the major risk factors for the various forms of dementia. Ginseng increases insulin sensitivity and reduces post-prandial glucose in animals. It has also been found to reduce inflammatory processes, such as levels of TNF-alpha in laboratory rats. In mice, ginsenosides block the effects of NF-κB, which is one of the major pro-inflammatory signals in the brain and other tissues. Ginseng may also reduce levels of cortisol, a major contributor to metabolic syndrome.

Chronic use of ginseng enhances insulin sensitivity in patients with diabetes type 2. An interesting observation is that application of ginseng extract to human cells causes effects similar to those of insulin. In studies using sheep cells, ginseng increases uptake of glucose into the cells, which is an effect that mimics insulin. Ginseng also stimulates release of insulin from the pancreas.

Ginseng has long been considered a tonic, restorative substance for the brain. In animal studies, ginsenosides have reduced inflammation in the brain and reduced amounts of beta amyloid in brain tissue. It has significant antioxidant activity. It has also been found to enhance neurogenesis in rat brains and appears to protect neurons from being triggered into apoptosis when subjected to overstimulation by the neurotransmitter glutamate. Ginseng does not affect cholinesterase enzymes, which is the mechanism of action of most of the prescribed medications dementia. However, there is evidence that it may enhance the brain's responsiveness to acetylcholine.

Long-term treatment of SAMP8 mice with ginseng has been found to significantly decrease the memory loss that is seen in these animals, which develop Alzheimer's-like lesions and loss of cognitive function as they age. Unfortunately, results have been inconsistent in the few studies in which ginseng was tested as a means to improve cognitive function in elderly and demented humans. In most cases, it has failed to provide discernible benefit. However, in one recent study published in the journal *Alzheimer Disease and Associated Disorders*, ginseng significantly improved the cognitive function of patients diagnosed with Alzheimer's dementia. Those benefits were seen over the twelve weeks of the experiment, as well as for several months after the experiment was ended. It is possible that in cases in which ginseng has been ineffective in patients with dementia, the treatment may have simply been too little, too late.

Overall, ginseng is a benign substance with no major adverse effects. Daily doses of 100 to 200 mg of standardized extract are generally very well tolerated. A little-appreciated fact is that ginsenosides have the basic molecular structure of steroids and some may exhibit estrogen-like effects in the body. A prudent caveat therefore is that women with a history of breast cancer should seek medical consent before starting daily treatment with ginseng.

GLYCERYLPHOSPHORYLCHOLINE

Glycerylphosphorylcholine (GPC) is yet another natural substance in the body. It serves primarily as a stepping stone in the biochemical pathways to produce other more important substances. If two fatty acid molecules are added to GCP, an easy trick for the brain's team of enzymes to perform, it becomes phosphatidylcholine. Phosphatidylcholine is an important component of cell membranes, as well as a primary source of choline. Choline in turn is used by the brain to produce the critical neurotransmitter acetylcholine. It is likely that GCP provides its benefits by being a raw material for phosphatidylcholine and acetylcholine. However, studies have shown that while GCP can be quite beneficial in the treatment of dementia, phosphatidylcholine is not. Thus, it is possible that GCP is more easily absorbed and utilized by the body, or that some hitherto unknown function of GCP gives it a unique ability to enhance cognitive function that phosphatidylcholine does not possess.

Most of what we know about the effects of GCP on brain chemistry and function comes from studies using laboratory animals. It has been found that GCP treatment increases the activity of the enzyme cholineacetyltransferase (ChAT), which is the enzyme responsible for the final step in producing acetylcholine. It is also found to increase the activity of acetylcholine in the hippocampus of aged rats. The hippocampus is an area of the brain of utmost importance in learning and memory, and we have long known that acetylcholine activity is diminished in the hippocampus and other areas of the brain in patients with Alzheimer's dementia. Most of the medications that are prescribed to treat Alzheimer's and other forms of dementia act by increasing the amount of acetylcholine in the brain. GCP treatment was also found to improve a characteristic of neuronal membranes called "fluidity." The normalization of membrane fluidity allows receptors for neurotransmitter signals to function properly. Yet another beneficial effect of GCP in rats was the ability to preserve neurons in the hippocampal structures of old rats that naturally develop high blood pressure. This condition would be similar to damage caused by high blood pressure in humans with vascular dementia of various types.

As would be expected from its effects on acetylcholine activity, GCP has been found to improve learning and memory in old rats that were showing deficits in such skills. GCP also improved cognitive deficits caused by treatment with the anticholinergic drug scopolamine. Anticholinergic medications are frequently found to cause confusion and cognitive deficits in elderly patients, including those who have not progressed to the point of being diagnosed with Alzheimer's dementia. It is interesting that GCP improved the cognitive function not only of old rats but, in some cases, young rats as well.

A number of studies performed over the past fifteen years have shown, with impressive consistency, that daily treatment with GCP in doses ranging from 600 to 1200 mg a day can improve cognitive function in patients suffering from a variety of conditions that lead to cognitive loss. These conditions have included mild cognitive impairment and Alzheimer's, vascular, and multi-infarct dementias. Effects have been seen as early as four weeks after initiating treatment. In at least one study, GCP was found to be as effective as the prescription medications Aricept and Exelon. I am not aware of any reports of significant adverse effects.

Because GCP almost certainly acts by increasing levels of phosphatidylcholine and acetylcholine, there is some question as whether it should be used with prescription medications for dementia that do the same, such as Razadyne, Aricept, or Exelon. In fact, because the mechanism by which it increases acetylcholinergic activity is different, it seems that GCP would complement and enhance the effects of these prescription medications rather than conflicting with them. There is a possibility of too much acetylcholinergic activity, which would likely manifest as nausea or other gastrointestinal upset, low heart rate, or nightmares. In any case, it is imperative to inform the prescribing physician about any plans to add GCP to a patient's medication regimen. It should be noted that the other prescription medication for dementia, memantine, does not act by increasing acetylcholinergic activity, thus there is less reason to suspect dangerous additive effects of GCP and memantine taken together. There is also a question as to whether GCP is redundant or additive to the effects of a similar substance, phosphatidylserine, which is available alone or in combination with other substances for treatment of dementia. The effects of phosphatidylserine and GCP may merely overlap, in which case using both would not be unreasonable. All in all, however, I would think that one or the other would be wiser and certainly cheaper than using both substances at the same time.

GRAPE SEED EXTRACT (PROCYANIDINS, PYCNOGENOL)

Grape skins and seeds contain a variety of complex biochemical substances that are increasingly being recognized as having a role in maintaining good health. One particularly interesting class of substances are the procyanidins, which are sometimes referred to as proanthocyanidins or Pycnogenol. The French biochemist Jacques Masquelier first extracted and identified procyanidins in 1936. He believed them to be so critical to human health that at first he referred to the procyanidins as "vitamin P." I suspect he was sorely disappointed when this name didn't catch on.

Procyanidins are polymers, or long molecular chains, built of simpler molecules called flavonoids. The flavonoids themselves offer many benefits, such as antioxidant and anti-inflammatory effects. It is not entirely clear if procyanidins are more beneficial than their component flavonoids are separately. In any case, a growing number of studies do show that procyanidins offer many benefits that would likely reduce the risk of dementia or improve function in patients already diagnosed with the illness.

Procyanidins in grape seed extracts are powerful antioxidants. In test tube studies, procyanidins were found to protect cells from the reactive oxygen species that are produced by the accumulation of beta amyloid. When cells were treated with procyanidins, they were less likely to suffer oxidation of fats in the cell membrane and had a decreased rate of being triggered into apoptosis, or programmed cell death. Treatment also blunted the inflammatory response stimulated by amyloid. In another study, procyanidins were as effective as vitamin E in protecting cells from amyloid toxicity. Similar protective effects of procyanidins in the brain were seen when live rats were given the substance by mouth. Along with decreasing oxidative damage to fat and protein, procyanidins also increased the activity of the neurotransmitter acetylcholine in the brains of those animals. Both of these effects would be of benefit to those at risk for Alzheimer's dementia.

Procyanidins also act to improve components of metabolic syndrome. They improve insulin sensitivity, and may even mimic some of insulin's beneficial effects. A favored way of inducing metabolic syndrome in laboratory animals is to feed them large amounts of sucrose or fructose. This causes insulin resistance, high blood pressure, and elevated triglycerides and cholesterol. However, when rats are given procyanidins along with the sugar, those manifestations of metabolic syndrome are significantly reduced. Procyanidins also appear to protect the brain from neurodegenerative effects of diabetes. High blood glucose levels damage the brain by allowing glucose molecules to unnaturally bind to proteins in brain cells. This abnormal process, called glycation, in turn triggers inflammatory responses. When diabetic rats are fed grape seed extracts, their brains are largely spared this damage. I am not aware of any large or definitive studies of effects of procyanidins on metabolic syndrome in humans. However, the data I have seen suggests that as in laboratory rats, it may help reduce cholesterol and triglycerides in our bodies as well.

The Tg2576 mouse is seen as a laboratory model of Alzheimer's dementia in humans. Feeding these animals grape seed extracts not only reduced the accumulation of beta amyloid in their brains, but also improved their learning and memory. There is only one report on the effect of procyanidins on cognitive function in healthy elderly humans. However, the effects in humans were quite similar to those seen in rodents. In this study, healthy men and women between the ages of sixty and eighty-five were given daily doses of 150 mg of procyanidins. After three months of treatment their memory functions were significantly improved.

Procyanidins can be obtained by that name, as grape seed extract, or as Pycnogenol. Pycnogenol is extracted from pine bark, but it is essentially the same substance as in grape seeds. The standard dose is 100 to 200 mg a day. To the best of my knowledge, there have been no reports of ill effects from the use of procyanidins from grape seed extract or other sources. Studies have been performed in mice to assess the safety of procyanidins, and doses equivalent to human use of 40 grams a day for six months were found to produce no ill effects. In view of the fact that such a dose is many times the usual recommended dose, there appears to be a wide margin of safety.

A good source of substances similar to procyanidins are berries, including blueberries, strawberries, blackberries, and raspberries. Studies using laboratory rats have shown that diets containing 2 percent blueberries can prevent and even reverse memory impairment that occurs in these animals as they age. Thus it appears that other colorfully hued fruits may share many of the same health benefits of grapes or grape seed extract.

GREEN TEA

Green tea is the product of one of several different ways to prepare the leaves of *Camellia sinensis*, which we commonly refer to as the tea plant. To make green tea, the leaves of the tea plant are steamed not long after being picked. This is in contrast to the process of making oolong and black teas, in which the leaves are allowed a long time to sit out and oxidize before being heated and dried. The method of preparing green tea maintains substantial quantities of a group of chemicals called catechins, particularly the substance epigallocatechin gallate (EGCG). Oolong and black teas have far less EGCG, due to oxidation. There is evidence that some of the chemicals that are produced in the oolong and black teas, such as theaflavins, can have benefits for health. However, green tea appears to be particularly helpful, and there are reports that consuming green tea can help prevent neurodegenerative dementias, including Alzheimer's and Lewy body dementias. Green tea has also been found to lower cholesterol, particularly the bad LDL form, decrease serum triglycerides, and improve the body's response to insulin. There are also reports that it can decrease blood pressure and inflammation.

Of particular interest are reports that the EGCG in green tea stimulates a physiological process called thermogenesis that leads the body to burn fat more rapidly and thereby helps people lose weight more readily. One way by which EGCG might do this is by inhibiting the enzymatic deactivation of adrenaline and noradrenaline. Those two substances can stimulate thermogenesis and contribute to weight loss and decrease in appetite. These indications that green tea can help in weight loss have been substantiated in several studies with human subjects. Together, existing data suggests that green tea can help combat metabolic syndrome and the obesity, diabetes, heart disease, and dementia that can result from it.

There are anecdotal reports of green tea helping concentration and cognitive function in humans; however, the only well-controlled scientific studies relevant to treating or preventing Alzheimer's dementia have been animal studies. Nonetheless, the data from animal studies has been very compelling. The catechins in green tea have been found to improve memory and learning in mice genetically engineered to suffer Alzheimer's-like changes in the brain. The EGCG of green tea reduces amyloid deposition in such mice. Catechins appear to both prevent production of amyloid protein as well as increase the activity of enzymes in the brain that break it down after it has formed. EGCG reduces inflammation, a major contributor to the progression of neurodegenerative diseases, by blunting the activity of two chemical triggers of inflammation, TNF-alpha and NF-κB. The substance also has a significant, albeit comparatively weak, ability to inhibit the destruction of the neurotransmitter acetylcholine in the brain. This is the mechanism of action of several drugs prescribed for the treatment of Alzheimer's dementia in humans. The catechins in green tea have antioxidant effects and appear to be able to grab iron from brain tissue and thus lower the tissue levels of this reactive metal. L-theanine, an unusual amino acid found in tea, has been found in both human and animal studies to have a calming effect without producing drowsiness. In animal studies, the substance appears to improve learning and memory.

Several cups of green tea a day should be sufficient to benefit from the catechins it contains. There is, however, a report from Japan that people who drank five cups of green tea per day, but not less than that, had a reduction in the likelihood of suffering a stroke. As there does not appear to be any ill effects of drinking green tea, it is not unreasonable to recommend two to five cups of this tea a day. It is also possible to obtain the benefits of green tea from capsules of tea extract. However, while this form of the herb appears to be relatively safe, there have been reports of liver damage in people taking large doses of concentrated extract of green tea. The U.S. Pharmacopeia studied the question of the safety of green tea extract, and they concluded that the product could be used safely, as long as people were warned not to abuse or misuse it.

HUPERZINE

Huperzine is extracted from the Chinese herb *Huperzia serrata*. The primary active component in huperzine is huperzine A. However, the herb also contains a variety of other active substances, including huperzine B, lycodine, lycodoline, serratine, serratinine, serratanidine, tohogenine, and other alkaloids that may be useful to treat human illness. In traditional Chinese medicine, the herb is known as "qian ceng ta," and for centuries it has been used to treat inflammation, fever, and swelling. In other parts of the world it is referred to as "Chinese club moss." Huperzine A is currently being evaluated in FDA-approved experiments to determine if it is a safe, effective treatment for dementia.

Huperzine is known to inhibit the breakdown of the neurotransmitter acetylcholine by the enzyme acetylcholinesterase, which is the mechanism of action of most of the medication approved by the FDA for treatment of dementia. However, it also appears able to reduce the toxic effects of too much glutamate. Glutamate "excitotoxicity" is one of the major causes of cell death in dementia. Overstimulation of damaged NMDA receptors, a subtype of glutamate receptor in the brain, allows leakage of calcium into neurons. This leakage of calcium damages neurons and adds "noise" to the processing of information in the brain. The prescription medication memantine acts by blocking abnormal glutamate stimulation of NMDA receptors. Huperzine also blocks abnormal activation of NMDA receptors in a manner very similar to that of memantine. Thus, huperzine appears to have multiple effects, two of which are the same as those of major prescribed medications. In addition, huperzine has been found to have antioxidant properties, anti-inflammatory effects, and an ability to stimulate dendritic growth of neurons. A particularly interesting finding is the recent report that huperzine A helps direct the processing of amyloid precursor protein into pathways that don't produce the sticky and dangerous forms of amyloid that accumulate as plaques in Alzheimer's dementia.

In studies using laboratory animals, huperzine has improved learning and memory and reduced microscopic evidence of neurodegenerative effects of amyloid. Huperzine has also been found to enhance learning in rats that have suffered reduction of blood flow to the brain, which is essentially an animal model of stroke or vascular dementia in humans. This improvement may be due in part to an ability of huperzine to increase production of BDNF and thus increase the rate of neurogenesis and neuron growth.

Numerous studies in China have shown huperzine to improve memory and other cognitive functions in human patients with Alzheimer's and vascular dementias, as well as what would be called MCI in the United States. In one of the first Chinese studies to reach Western audiences, an eight-week course of 200 mcg of huperzine A led to improvements in memory and other cognitive functions in nearly 60 percent of Alzheimer's patients participating in the study. A comprehensive battery of laboratory tests found no obvious ill effects of the treatment. In a 2008 study at the Mount Sinai College of Medicine, it was found that 200 mcg of huperzine a day was ineffective. However, 400 mcg per day of huperzine improved some aspects of cognitive function in patients already diagnosed with Alzheimer's dementia. The Cochrane reviewers have found that huperzine is promising. However, in their most recent report on the subject, in 2008, they did not yet feel that enough studies had been done for them to give wholehearted support to the use of the substance for treatment of dementia. If and when huperzine enters the FDA's phase III trials, in which large-scale human studies would be performed, we should gain a clearer understanding of its effectiveness.

At present it can be said that huperzine has the same mechanisms of action as existing medications prescribed for dementia, and that it has been found in preliminary studies in both China and the United States to improve memory and cognitive function in some patients with Alzheimer's dementia. It has few side effects and is safe for elderly individuals to use on a daily basis for at least several months at a time.

IBUPROFEN

Ibuprofen is something of an odd duck in this section. It is not an herb, vitamin, or "nutraceutical." Until not too many years ago, ibuprofen was a prescription medication available only by your doctor's order. It can have serious side effects in some people, and it must therefore be approached in a serious manner. Ibuprofen is serious medicine. I have included it because it is a readily available, inexpensive medication that can be purchased over-the-counter without need of a doctor's prescription. There is substantial evidence that daily use of ibuprofen can help reduce the risk of Alzheimer's dementia. Perhaps most importantly, there is clear indication that a lot of people are already using ibuprofen in hopes of avoiding Alzheimer's dementia.

Ibuprofen is a medication used to treat mild pain and inflammation. It is in a class of medications known as non-steroidal anti-inflammatory drugs or NSAIDs. NSAIDs are thought to work by preventing the production of prostaglandins in the body. There are many different types of prostaglandins. In many respects they act as hormones. However, unlike hormones such as insulin or thyroxine, which are released into the blood to organize and synchronize metabolic activity throughout the body, prostaglandins are designed to act more locally. Cells stimulated to produce prostaglandins release them into the tissue that surrounds them, where they help alter various types of physiological activities in the cells in the immediate vicinity. Some prostaglandins increase inflammatory responses, and others dampen them. They do a variety of important jobs in the body, and it is safe to say that their many roles are essential for good health. Prostaglandins are simply the messengers of information and are not themselves good or bad. However, when injury of some kind has occurred, certain prostaglandins stimulate processes of pain and swelling of which we often wish to rid ourselves. Prostaglandins can also mediate some of the damaging effects of oxidative stress, AGEs, and other sources of inflammatory processes in the brain.

Ibuprofen is one of many NSAIDs that block the activity of the enzyme cyclooxygenase (COX). This is where things get complicated and controversial. There are two types of COX, known as COX-1 and COX-2. Ibuprofen blocks both types of the enzyme. The drugs Viiox and Celebrex, which have been the focus of so much concern in the press, specifically inhibit COX-2. In 2004, after enjoying tremendous success in its ability to relieve pain and discomfort in individuals who had not previously found relief from their symptoms, Viiox was yanked from the market after it was found to increase the risk of heart disease, stroke, and sudden cardiac death. Soon afterward, Celebrex was also found to increase the risk of cardiac death. It was as if a bomb had dropped. Controversy has subsequently arisen over whether or not ibuprofen and similar NSAIDs also increase the risk of cardiac death. Results have been inconsistent, which suggests that the risk may depend upon the history of the patient. It appears that people who have already been diagnosed with heart disease face a slightly higher risk of progression of the disease and cardiac death if they take ibuprofen or certain other NSAIDs. Moreover, it appears that this effect is dose-dependent, that is, the higher the doses of ibuprofen, the higher the risk.

The relevance of ibuprofen to this book is that since the connection was first reported in 1996, it has been clearly established that people who have taken ibuprofen daily over many years to treat conditions such as arthritis have a significantly reduced risk of developing Alzheimer's dementia. A study as recent as 2008 from the Boston University School of Medicine showed that chronic use of ibuprofen for five years or more reduces the risk of Alzheimer's by half. Of particular interest is the fact that while this effect of ibuprofen has been attributed to its anti-inflammatory effects, not all NSAIDs have been shown to reduce the risk of Alzheimer's in the same way as ibuprofen. This has led scientists to suspect that ibuprofen may have some effects other than blocking COX enzymes that may help reduce the risk of dementia. In fact, ibuprofen is able to reduce the amount of the sticky form of amyloid protein, called ABeta42, probably by affecting the way the enzyme gamma secretase processes amyloid precursor protein. Ibuprofen also decreases levels of the sticky form of amyloid by stimulating a messenger in the cell called PPAR. Interestingly, PPAR is also stimulated by insulin, and it mediates many of insulin's most important effects. Some drugs that stimulate PPAR are used to treat diabetes, and are known to be beneficial in treating metabolic syndrome. To the best of my knowledge there are no reports of ibuprofen having any benefits for relieving metabolic syndrome in humans. However, there is a report that it can prevent the progression of metabolic syndrome into diabetes type 2 in laboratory rats. It is interesting that ibuprofen does not appear to block cholinesterase enzymes or activity at the NMDA receptors, which are the main mechanisms of action of the FDA-approved medications for treating dementia. Thus, ibuprofen may act by unique mechanisms to reduce the risk of dementia. This is important because it means that the effects of ibuprofen could be additive to the effects of standard medications in the prevention and treatment of the condition.

In *Goodman and Gilman's The Pharmacological Basis of Therapeutics*, one of the bibles of medical practice, it is noted that nearly 15 percent of patients started on ibuprofen by their doctors have to discontinue it because of side effects that may include stomach pain, heartburn, and nausea. Like other NSAIDs, ibuprofen can cause bleeding in the stomach, although this happens less often than is seen with the NSAID aspirin. *Goodman and Gilman's* also recommends that ibuprofen not be used by women who are pregnant or nursing. I strongly recommend that you discuss any plans to start daily treatment with ibuprofen with your doctor. No one with a history of heart disease should consider it.

IDEBENONE

Idebenone is a synthetic substance that can serve as a replacement for the natural substance co-enzyme Q10. CoQ10 plays a critical role in the electron transport chain, which is the molecular assembly line in mitochondria that produces the energy-storing molecule ATP. ATP is the source of chemical energy that powers cells in all their activities. All cells, regardless of what they do or where they are in the body, require ATP to live and function. Along with helping to produce ATP in the mitochondria, CoQ10 also plays a protective role by acting as an antioxidant. The chemical process that produces ATP, called oxidative phosphorylation, consists of a series of very high-energy reactions that unavoidably produce reactive oxygen species (ROS) as by-products. ROS molecules attack other molecules and oxidize them. Oxidation can destroy necessary molecules, cause buildup of tangles of indigestible lipofuscin in the cell, interfere with chemical processes and insulin sensitivity, and trigger inflammation. When ROS molecules are loose in a cell, chemical alarms sound, and the cell pulls out all the stops to bring the situation back under control. CoQ10 and other antioxidants in the cell help keep the levels of ROS molecules in check. They not only limit the amount of oxidative damage, but they also prevent the cell from having to go into emergency mode.

Idebenone can substitute for CoQ10 in the electron transport chain, where it works perfectly well in producing ATP. Idebenone is also a powerful antioxidant. However, there are some important differences between idebenone and CoQ10. In the past ten years or so, it has been found that CoQ10 has a quirk that manifests when oxygen levels in the body get low. Under conditions of low oxygen, instead of helping to neutralize ROS molecules, CoQ10 actually helps to create more ROS. Instead of acting as an antioxidant, CoQ10 becomes a pro-oxidant. Although this seems counterintuitive, the reason CoQ10 acts in this way can be explained. An ongoing lack of oxygen is a rare but dire emergency for a cell, and it must quickly marshal all of its resources to change the situation or at least adapt to weather the storm. The pro-oxidant effect of CoQ10 in hypoxic states takes advantage of the extreme response the cell has to ROS molecules. Thus, CoQ10 is used to produce ROS as a means of pulling the "fire alarm." Although yelling "fire" in a flood is a peculiar thing to do, it still gets everyone's attention, which is the desired result. Unfortunately, there are some conditions in which states of low oxygen in specific tissues or throughout the body become chronic. When hypoxia is chronic, the extreme response to the drop in oxygen itself becomes chronic, and the inflammation and increased oxidation become additional chronic sources of tissue damage. When this occurs in the brain, the damage can lead to dementia. Unlike CoQ10, idebenone continues to function as an antioxidant in states of hypoxia. It does not stimulate production of ROS. Moreover, instead of being hijacked to oxidize molecules and set off the ROS alarm, idebenone can continue on with the necessary work of producing ATP. In conditions that include sleep apnea, chronic obstructive pulmonary disease, congestive heart failure, stroke, and vascular dementia, there are distinct advantages to having a significant level of idebenone in the body to help prevent oxidative damage and maintain metabolism.

Along with acting as an antioxidant, idebenone also has anti-inflammatory effects. Although less potent than NSAIDs such as ibuprofen, it can inhibit the enzymes cyclooxygenase and lipoxygenase, which turn the fatty acid arachidonic acid into inflammatory substances called eicosanoids. Idebenone has been found to prevent impairment of learning and memory in rats that have had amyloid protein injected into their brains, and this may be due to its antioxidant and anti-inflammatory effects. Of particular interest are reports that idebenone stimulates nerve growth factor (NGF) in the brain. Administration of idebenone has been found to increase levels of NGF in the brain tissue of old rats and to restore production of acetylcholine and normal behavior in the brains of rats that had had damage done to the basal forebrain. The basal forebrain is an area that contains neurons that produce and release acetylcholine, levels of which decrease in the brains of patients with Alzheimer's dementia.

A surprisingly large number of studies have been performed to test the effects of idebenone on the cognitive function of people with dementia. In a few studies, idebenone was found to be of no benefit in patients with Alzheimer's dementia. However, in the vast majority of scientific studies, idebenone did improve or at least help maintain cognitive function in patients with mild to moderate Alzheimer's dementia. These benefits were found to continue for as long as two years of treatment. In one case, idebenone was found to be as effective as tacrine, a drug that is FDA-approved but now rarely used for the treatment of Alzheimer's dementia. Idebenone also improves cognitive function in vascular dementia, which may be due in part to its ability to maintain activity in the electron transport chain without increasing oxidative stress during periods of hypoxia. At least one study looked for benefits in using idebenone to treat patients with mild cognitive impairment, but no benefits were observed. A wide range of doses of idebenone have been found to be effective in treating dementia. The lowest effective dose, which has been used in several successful studies, appears to be 90 mg a day. No study, even the few in which idebenone was ineffective, found the substance to have toxic effects in doses ranging from 90 mg to 720 mg a day. Idebenone is available in some health food stores and on the Internet.

LEMON BALM

Lemon balm, officially known as *Melissa officinalis*, is a member of the mint family that has a long history of use as a calming and restorative herb. It has been thought to relieve anxiety, improve sleep, lift mood, and sharpen memory. In her *Modern Herbal*, the estimable M. (Margaret) Grieve notes that the great Paracelsus held lemon balm in high regard, believing that it could "completely revivify a man." She also refers to a statement by the herbalist John Evelyn who wrote, "Balm is sovereign for the brain, strengthening the memory and powerfully chasing away melancholy."

Modern scientific techniques have confirmed that lemon balm has pharmacological properties that could make it effective in addressing some of the neurochemical imbalances that occur in dementia. However, the strength and consistency of these effects tend to be overstated. Some studies have shown that lemon balm contains substances that block acetylcholinesterase, which in turn would raise levels of the neurotransmitter acetylcholine in the brain. This is the mechanism of action of the medications most often prescribed for Alzheimer's dementia. It also has the ability to mimic acetylcholine and stimulate several types of acetylcholine receptors in the brain. Indeed, substances in lemon balm have modest affinity for two of the major types of acetylcholine receptors in brain tissue, that is, nicotinic and muscarinic receptors. Like sage, rosemary, and a number of other aromatic herbs, lemon balm contains antioxidants and rosmarinic acid, which has been found to buffer against some of the toxic effects of amyloid in the brain.

In the earliest study of the effects of lemon balm on cognitive function, extracts of the herb actually impaired the performance of healthy young adults. It was suspected that the method of preparing lemon balm for this study led to the retention of sedating properties of the herb but none of the properties that might lead to sharpening of attention and memory. When exacting scientific methods were used in a subsequent study to confirm the presence of cholinergic components, that is, substances that mimicked acetylcholine, improvements in both calmness and cognitive function were observed. However, whereas the extracts of lemon balm were found to have modest effects at acetylcholine receptors, they were found to have no ability to block the enzyme cholinesterase. In a study of patients already diagnosed with Alzheimer's dementia, four months of treatment with lemon balm produced significant improvements in cognitive function and decreases in agitation.

The most impressive results from the evaluations of lemon balm on cognitive function and mood are that improvements can be seen with no indications of toxicity. However, while calming effects are consistently reported, the effects on cognitive function vary. Even in the hands of experts, there seems to be significant variation in what substances and pharmacological properties can be found in any one preparation. This may be due to variables as simple as when and where the plants were grown, freshness of samples, and certainly how the medicinal properties were extracted form plant material. Although further research may reveal methods to more accurately predict properties and effects of preparations of lemon balm, it would be imprudent at this time to recommend the herb as an effective and dependable method for the prevention or treatment of such a serious illness as Alzheimer's dementia. Nonetheless, the herb is harmless and compatible with other likely more potent treatments. It does have calming effects as well as antioxidants and rosmarinic acid. If you enjoy the lemony flavor and aroma of lemon balm tea, then by all means use it. Grieve points out that the fresh leaves make a better tea than the dry; moreover, they are likely to better provide any beneficial medicinal properties as well.

MELATONIN

Melatonin is a hormone that is natural to the body. It is produced by the pineal gland, a small gland that sits in the center of the brain. The name "pineal" is derived from the fact that it has a shape reminiscent of a tiny pine cone. The pineal gland enjoys a certain notoriety for having been suspected by the famous French philosopher and mathematician Rene Descartes to be the site at which the human soul interacts with the brain. He suspected this because the pineal gland is the only structure in the brain that is central, single, and solitary, without being split into two symmetrical lobes as are the cerebral cortex and other major structures. Descartes believed that since the soul is the source of human consciousness and the mirror of the divine, one true God, it could not possibly sit across divided structures of the brain. The pineal gland appeared to be the only place in which the seat of the soul could reasonably exist in the human brain.

The primary role of melatonin is to serve as one of the time-keeping substances in the body, helping synchronize the body's activities with the day and night cycle of the environment. The cyclic changes in the body that occur daily as day goes to night are called circadian rhythms. Melatonin is able to synchronize the body with the environment because the pineal gland releases the hormone according to information that is relayed to it from the eyes by way of the sympathetic nervous system. During the day, when sunlight is falling on the retina in the back of the eye, the production and release of melatonin is inhibited. At dusk, as the sun begins to drop in the sky, the pineal gland is released from inhibition and begins to produce and release melatonin into the bloodstream. Melatonin helps the brain prepare for nighttime, and it is known to be part of the system that allows the mind and brain to fall asleep. Melatonin is available over the counter as a sleep aid, and a new medication, Rozerem, which mimics some of the effects of melatonin on the brain, can be prescribed by doctors for certain individuals who are bothered by insomnia.

Melatonin production by the pineal gland decreases with age. The most dramatic decreases in melatonin production are seen about the age of sixty. For reasons that aren't yet understood, this decrease in melatonin is more apparent in men than in women. Of interest is the now well-established finding that people who suffer Alzheimer's dementia have far lower levels of melatonin in their blood than do people of the same age who do not suffer the illness. It is possible that Alzheimer's dementia damages the brain and thus causes deficits in the production of melatonin. However, it has long been suspected that low levels of melatonin may somehow contribute to the pathological processes of Alzheimer's.

Melatonin has a number of effects in the brain that would be expected to help prevent Alzheimer's dementia. Melatonin is a powerful antioxidant and scavenger of reactive oxygen species that damage brain tissue and stimulate inflammatory responses. It also stimulates the activation of enzymes such as superoxide dismutase and glutathione reductase, which provide further protection from oxidative stress. It may even block inflammation directly, in much the same way that ibuprofen does.

Melatonin not only protects brain cells from the toxic effects of amyloid, it also helps prevent formation of sticky sheets of amyloid that form into plaques in the brain. Melatonin also increases levels of neural growth factors and blocks the inhibition of neurogenesis by the stress hormone cortisol. Together, these effects of melatonin help maintain brain tissue. Melatonin protects against oxidative damage in Parkinson's disease and buffers against a phenomenon known as excitotoxic damage in the brain, which occurs when the blood supply is cut off, such as would occur in a stroke. Melatonin improves glucose tolerance and improves insulin sensitivity. Thus, along with dampening some of the primary degenerative processes underlying Alzheimer's and other dementias, melatonin may provide protection from a variety of problems that often lead to dementia.

In one interesting study, mice that had been given human genes for amyloid and that tend to develop the same amyloid plaques seen in Alzheimer's were treated with melatonin. The transgenic mice that received melatonin were slower to develop amyloid plaques in their brains, and they lived longer than the mice that did not receive melatonin. This may be due to melatonin reducing production of amyloid itself. Melatonin is known to help improve the behavior of patients with Alzheimer's and in particular to reduce the phenomenon of "sundowning" that is so often seen in this group of patients. Sundowning is an increase in confusion, agitation, and even aggressive behaviors that occurs in the early evening as sundown approaches. Melatonin does not improve cognitive functions in patients with Alzheimer's, but it may slow the loss of cognitive functions. There is a fascinating report of a pair of identical twins who both developed Alzheimer's dementia. One of them was started on daily treatment with melatonin, whereas the other twin was not. After three years, the twin who received the melatonin had substantially better memory and other cognitive functions than the twin who did not receive melatonin. Still, it is not yet known if a lack of melatonin can actually cause Alzheimer's or other forms of dementia, or if maintaining normal levels of melatonin can help prevent dementia.

Overall, melatonin is natural and appears quite safe. It is readily available as an over-the-counter medication. However, the purity and quantity of the melatonin found in such preparations can vary considerably. I have been told by an expert in sleep medicine who has studied the effects of melatonin that some over-the-counter bottles labeled as "melatonin" have been analyzed for dose and purity and found not to contain *any* of the substance. Thus, it is imperative that a pharmacist or another trusted individual be consulted about the best brands of melatonin to purchase.

PHOSPHATIDYLSERINE

Phosphatidylserine is a building block of the fatty membrane that surrounds and contains every cell in the body. It serves an important role in the structure and function of neurons, and it is found in particularly high concentration in the brain. Phosphatidylserine molecules are positioned in the inner layer of the cell membrane and usually cannot be detected on the outer layer of the cell that comes into contact with other cells in that tissue or with immune cells that may pass by while doing their "surveillance" of the body. When phosphatidylserine does end up on the outer layer of a normal cell, a special enzyme called "flipase" flips the phosphatidylserine back into its normal position in the inner layer. When cells are damaged, primarily by oxidative stress, phosphatidylserine can end up permanently on the outside surface of the cell.

The misplacement of phosphatidylserine into the outer membrane triggers within the cell the process of cellular suicide called apoptosis. The phosphatidylserine on the outer membrane then serves as a marker of a damaged cell that is dying and needs to be "eaten" by a macrophage. Unfortunately, individuals with Alzheimer's dementia tend to lose the normal, asymmetrical positioning of phosphatidylserine in the inner layer of the cell membranes of neurons, which is likely to contribute to destruction of neurons in the brain. Although phosphatidylserine may seem to be contributing to the damage by raising the cell's "eat me" flag, it actually serves the critical function of helping the cell go quietly and without causing a disturbance in the cellular neighborhood. In fact, when macrophages sense the presence of phosphatidylserine on the outside of a cell, they turn off their inflammatory processes before they sit down to dine on the unfortunate cell. Without sufficient phosphatidylserine, the inflammatory processes generated by dying cells would more seriously damage tissue.

Along with having anti-inflammatory effects, phosphatidylserine is also an antioxidant. Old mice that had been given genes that produce an Alzheimer's-like disease in those animals are found to have reduced levels of phosphatidylserine in the cell membranes of their neurons. Phosphatidylserine treatment helps prevent the inflammation and damage that amyloid protein deposits can cause in the brain tissue of such animals. There is also evidence that a lack of sufficient phosphatidylserine in the cells that line blood vessels increases inflammation due to the sheer stress of blood rushing past them. Thus, supplementation can help prevent vascular problems that contribute to both Alzheimer's and vascular dementia. Phosphatidylserine increases the release of acetylcholine from brain tissue of old rats and thus mimics some of the effects of the major medications prescribed for Alzheimer's dementia in humans. In old rats, phosphatidylserine also increases the dendritic branching of neurons in the brain, which allows them to process information more effectively.

A substantial number of studies have been performed in humans that show that treatment with phosphatidylserine may help prevent, delay, or alleviate some symptoms of Alzheimer's dementia. The vast majority of studies have shown that in patients diagnosed with Alzheimer's dementia, 300 to 400 mg of phosphatidylserine a day slows the loss of cognitive function. In some studies there have actually been some minor improvements in function, which is a result rarely seen even with prescribed medications. People with MCI who had not yet progressed to the diagnosis of Alzheimer's dementia showed improvement in their cognitive function over a twelve-week period of receiving 300 mg of phosphatidylserine a day. Thus, treatment may help prevent or delay the progression from MCI to outright dementia. Doses of phosphatidylserine as large as 600 mg a day have been found to be entirely without ill effects in otherwise healthy individuals. It is not known if adults who are free of cognitive losses can in any way benefit from supplementing with phosphatidylserine.

RED YEAST RICE

Red yeast rice is produced by cultivating the growth of a brilliantly colored red yeast called *Monascus purpureus* on ordinary white rice. Red yeast rice, which is referred to by the Chinese as "ang khak" and by the Japanese as "koji," has been used in the Orient for centuries as both a food and a medicine. Descriptions of the use of red yeast rice as a treatment for digestive disturbances and as a general tonic appear in Chinese writings dating as far back as the first century AD. Of particular interest is the fact that some of the substances produced in the fermentation activity of *Monascus purpureus* are active in reducing the synthesis of cholesterol in the human body. In fact, those specific substances, and likely other biochemicals in red yeast rice, appear to produce a variety of beneficial effects that would be expected to reduce the risk of cardiovascular disease, metabolic syndrome, diabetes, and dementia.

Among the many by-products of the metabolism of *Monascus purpureus* yeast are a group of biochemicals called monacolins. There are at least nine different monacolins in red yeast rice, and they are likely to be responsible for many of its salutary effects. Indeed, one of these monacolins, called monacolin K, is identical to the drug lovastatin. Lovastatin was marketed by the Merck pharmaceutical company as the first so-called statin drug to treat high cholesterol. As might be expected from its containing lovastatin, extracts of red yeast rice have been found to reduce both bad LDL cholesterol and triglycerides in human subjects, without affecting levels of the good HDL cholesterol. One such study of the effects of red yeast rice was published in the *American Journal of Clinical Nutrition*. In that study it was noted that substances other than the lovastatin in red yeast rice likely contributed to its cholesterol-lowering effect. Red yeast rice does contain substances known as phytosterols, which prevent the passage of cholesterol from the intestine into the bloodstream. These phytosterols might thus enhance the cholesterol-lowering effects of red yeast rice. In Chinese studies, red yeast rice has been found to increase insulin sensitivity in human subjects with diabetes type 2. In animal studies, it was found to act like insulin in decreasing the production of glucose by the liver, which would explain the beneficial effects seen in the diabetic patients. These effects of red yeast rice would be expected to help prevent metabolic syndrome and the many problems that can arise from that condition, including dementia.

The statin class of medications is starting to be seen as having many beneficial effects beyond simply helping to treat hypercholesterolemia. Current evidence suggests that statins reduce the risk of dementia not only by improving serum cholesterol and triglyceride levels, but also by acting as antioxidants, reducing the production of beta amyloid, and dampening the damaging inflammatory effects of amyloid in brain tissue. Although statins have not been recognized by the FDA as a means to prevent or treat Alzheimer's and other forms of dementia, this class of drugs is more and more being seen as a means to reduce the risk of developing those illnesses. My understanding is that there are papers written in Chinese showing that red yeast rice may be of benefit in reducing the risk of dementia, but I have not personally seen solid scientific evidence of such benefit. There are, however, several interesting studies showing positive effects of red yeast rice in animal models of Alzheimer's dementia. In one case, red yeast rice prevented deterioration of memory in rats that had had sticky forms of amyloid protein injected into their brains. Interestingly, the red yeast rice was more effective in protecting the cognitive function of these rats than was lovastatin, which suggests that lovastatin isn't the only substance in red yeast rice that could help prevent progression of Alzheimer's dementia. Red yeast rice was also found to prevent inflammatory and oxidative damage caused by amyloid in the brain and to prevent the deposition of amyloid protein into the plaques that damage brain tissue.

In studies of red yeast rice in humans, the effective doses tend to range from 1 to 3 grams per day. One gram of red yeast rice contains approximately 2 mg of lovastatin. The usual starting dose of lovastatin is 20 mg a day, which again points to the likelihood of substances other than lovastatin contributing to the beneficial effects of red yeast rice. Unfortunately, this product is not under FDA control or supervision, and the purity and concentration of the medicinal components of the red yeast rice cannot always be guaranteed. If you pursue treatment with red yeast rice, it is advisable to purchase a reputable brand from a dealer you know and trust. I certainly wouldn't use some product advertised at a cheap price on the Internet.

Most reports suggest that red yeast rice is safe and well tolerated, and many experts insist that it is safer than statins. Such a belief seems consistent with the fact that it has been used for centuries in the Orient as a food and condiment. In a study published in the journal *Current Therapeutic*

Research, subjects enjoyed significant decreases in serum cholesterol and triglycerides with the only adverse effects being a few complaints of flatulence, dizziness, and heartburn. Therapeutic doses do not appear to harm the liver or kidneys. Still, red yeast rice, like statins, should be seen as a potentially dangerous substance. I note, for example, that a renal transplant patient was reported to experience a potentially lethal case of rhabdomyolysis while taking red yeast rice. Rhabdomyolysis is a dangerous disturbance of muscle metabolism that can affect the kidneys and other organs. It can be caused by treatment with statins, and prudent doctors monitor their patients receiving these medicines for symptoms of rhabdomyolysis (particularly muscle pain and fatigue) to prevent the rare but potentially lethal condition. The unfortunate case I mentioned above was most likely due to anti–organ rejection medication interacting in a peculiar way with the red yeast rice. Nonetheless, the case illustrates the fact that natural substances that are powerful enough to help you are also powerful enough to hurt you under certain circumstances. If you plan on taking red yeast rice, first inform your doctor. Note that experts advise against the use of red yeast rice in individuals who are pregnant, nursing, or suffering liver or kidney impairment; patients who are already taking a statin drug, niacin, or gemfibrozil for high cholesterol; or people receiving the medications cyclosporin, azole antifungals, erythromycin, clarithromycin, nefazodone, or protease inhibitors. Stay away from grapefruit juice, as it prevents the metabolism of statins. As is the case with prescribed statin medications, red yeast rice would be expected to inhibit the synthesis of co-enzyme Q10 to some degree. Thus, if you take red yeast rice, you should supplement with CoQ10.

RESVERATROL

The term "The French Paradox" refers to the fact that despite their love of pastries, gravies, and rich, high-calorie foods, the French have a surprisingly low rate of heart disease. It has long been suspected that the bottle of red wine, ever present on the French dinner table, may have something to do with their apparent resistance to the effects of imprudent diet. There is evidence that moderate consumption of red wine may also help reduce the risk of dementia.

Wine is a complicated mix of alcohol and a variety of plant-derived substances that give the wine color and flavor. Any one of those substances could, in addition, provide health benefits. One substance in red wine that may contribute to its beneficial effects is resveratrol. Resveratrol is one of several multi-ringed molecules called polyphenols, which are produced in grapes and other food plants in response to fungus infections and environmental stresses. I recall an interesting comment in the literature about the suspicion that the chemicals used in modern agriculture decrease the amount of resveratrol and similar substances in our food. Ostensibly, this would be due to the plants not needing to produce resveratrol, as they are no longer beset by natural diseases from which they would need to protect themselves. Thus, an extra benefit of eating organic produce is that aside from being free of potentially dangerous chemicals, it may be richer in resveratrol and related substances.

An extraordinary range of health benefits have been attributed to resveratrol. There is compelling evidence that resveratrol may help prevent or control cardiovascular and metabolic conditions that are risk factors for dementia. In animal studies, resveratrol has been found to reduce the deposition of fat in the lining of arteries, lower high blood pressure, and reduce the release of inflammatory substances from fat cells that surround the gut. Resveratrol has been found to reduce insulin resistance, which would reduce the risk of metabolic syndrome and diabetes. Resveratrol is thus thought to contribute to the ability of red wine to reduce the risk of metabolic syndrome, cardiovascular disease, and diabetes. However, these hypotheses remain to be proven by scientific study.

One of the most remarkable effects attributed to resveratrol is an ability to extend the length of life itself. When animals are restricted in their calorie intake, they tend to live longer. This appears to be the case over a wide range of species, from worms to mammals. Calorie restriction stimulates the activity of a protein called SIR-2, which is thought to be at least partially responsible for the increase in longevity. Resveratrol enhances the activity of SIR-2 in yeast cells, extending their life span. Resveratrol also extends the life span of worms, fruit flies, and, most recently, it has been found to lengthen the life of a small vertebrate fish. Preliminary reports have suggested that resveratrol may also increase the life span of mammals, specifically, the mouse. In test tube studies, resveratrol stimulates the activity of a human analog of SIR-2, known as SIRT-1. Thus, there is reason to suspect that resveratrol may produce some of these same life-extending effects in humans.

There are many effects of resveratrol in brain tissue that could be expected to reduce the risk of dementia. Resveratrol is a powerful antioxidant, and in test tube studies it has been found to protect brain cells from the neurotoxic effects of amyloid. Those neurotoxic effects are at least partially due to oxidative damage. Resveratrol also improves the energy output of mitochondria in brain cells exposed to amyloid and reduces the likelihood of them dying by apoptosis. Other studies have found that resveratrol blocks some of the inflammatory effects of amyloid in brain tissue. It appears to do so by dampening the activity of NF-κB, which is one of the primary triggers of the inflammatory response.

When given to living mice genetically engineered to develop a condition similar to Alzheimer's dementia as they age, resveratrol reduced the burden of amyloid plaque in their brain tissue. That effect was explained as being due to the ability of resveratrol to help break down and remove amyloid after it has been deposited. If that is indeed the case, then resveratrol might be useful in reversing symptoms of cognitive dysfunction in individuals who have already acquired a burden of amyloid plaque in their brains. Perhaps most importantly, a recent study performed in China found that treating with resveratrol improved cognitive function in mice that develop an Alzheimer's-like condition.

An argument against resveratrol being an important component of red wine's effects, or even a practical treatment in its own right, is that it has extremely low bioavailability. Bioavailability is a measure of how much of a substance is actually available inside an animal to bring about effects. About 70 percent of ingested resveratrol gets into the human bloodstream, which is a reasonably high absorption rate. However, little if any of the pure resveratrol remains in the blood after what is absorbed from the intestine makes its first pass through the liver. Thus, it is difficult to understand how even fairly high doses of resveratrol could do anything of significance if ingested by real, living human beings. In any case, if you enjoy drinking moderate amounts of red wine, then keep doing it. There are many other polyphenols in wine other than resveratrol that probably do get absorbed and distributed in the body in helpful concentrations. If the small amount of resveratrol in the wine is adding to your health, then so much the better. On the other hand, until a process or route of administration is devised to increase the bioavailability of resveratrol, I would not spend money on resveratrol tablets to supplement your intake.

As a final caveat, recent studies have suggested that while resveratrol may extend life expectancy, its effects on the brain may not be entirely beneficial. SIRT-1 activity may prolong life in part by repairing damaged DNA and preventing cells from dying by apoptosis. Resveratrol is known to activate SIRT-1. In the brain, SIRT-1 can also be stimulated by inflammation and oxidative damage. One effect of SIRT-1 in the damaged brain is to push neural stem cells that might ordinarily become neurons into becoming cells known as astrocytes. Astrocytes do not process information, rather they act like custodians, standing guard over brain tissue and cleaning up when tissue is damaged. It is overproduction of astrocytes that is largely responsible for scarring in spinal cord injury. Similar disruption of function, perhaps dementia, can occur in the brain when SIRT-1 drives neural progenitor cells into becoming astrocytes rather than evolving into neurons through the process of neurogenesis. As a final thought, while the normal liver readily destroys the resveratrol in red wine, and thus protects the brain from any potential ill effects of this substance, a liver severely damaged by years of alcoholism might not. I wonder if over-consumption of resveratrol might contribute to the dreaded neurodegenerative Marchiafava-Bignami disease, which, on rare occasion, afflicts chronic abusers of large quantities of red wine.

RHODIOLA

Rhodiola rosea is an herb that grows in the northern climes of Asia. Its medicinal effects have been appreciated since ancient times, and it has been used in folk medicines of Russia and Scandinavia for many years. The herb has gone largely unrecognized in the United States. However, largely due to the work of Dr. Richard Brown, a Columbia University physician well versed in herbal medicine and other alternative modes of treatment, rhodiola is coming to be seen as a useful and possibly important herbal supplement. Brown, who has written extensively on the benefits and uses of rhodiola, has noted that in many traditional folk medicines, rhodiola has been seen as a herb for revitalizing the body and improving concentration, strength, and endurance. Following the lead of Russian researchers, who have done the lion's share of the technical studies on the pharmacology and use of rhodiola, Brown refers to the herb as an "adaptogen." He defines adaptogen as a substance that provides an overall enhancement of the body's resistance to stress. He has emphasized that the name rhodiola refers to a large number of related species, but the plant *Rhodiola rosea* is specifically endowed with health benefits, and it is this particular species about which we have the most information. My references to rhodiola should thus be taken to mean specifically *Rhodiola rosea*. Rhodiola contains a number of active substances collectively known as rosavins, which remain active after extraction from the plant. But, as Brown fully admits, it is not yet known exactly which components of rhodiola are responsible for its beneficial effects.

There is evidence that Rhodiola enhances the synthesis and release of various neurotransmitters in the brain. It also has strong antioxidant effects.

In animal studies, rhodiola has enhanced learning and memory. In human studies, the herb has been found to improve attention, performance, memory, and learning, particularly in cases in which the adverse effects of overwork and fatigue would have set in. For example, in a test of performance in proofreading text, a notoriously difficult challenge of one's capacity to stay on task despite the long, tedious, and mind-numbing necessity for attention to minor detail, readers who had been given rhodiola prior to the task performed with far fewer errors over an eight-hour period. The herb is found to help relieve a variety of physical complaints that often occur in the context of overwork, depression, and anxiety, such as irritability, distractibility, fatigue, headache, and weakness.

There are substances in rhodiola that inhibit the activity of the enzyme cholinesterase in the brain. This effect would increase activity of the neurotransmitter acetylcholine, and this is the same mechanism of action of the majority of the medications prescribed by physicians to treat dementia. Salidroside, a substance found in rhodiola, is able to reduce the oxidative damage caused by exposure of brain cells to amyloid protein. When extracts of rhodiola are given to rats prior to causing them severe stress by keeping them immobilized, the unwillingness to eat that such animals generally show afterward is prevented. This effect of rhodiola was probably due to an ability to blunt the effects of the stress response, as it also prevented the expected lack of appetite after corticotrophin releasing hormone (CRH) was microinjected directly into their brains. CRH is one of the first chemical triggers in the brain's response to stress. It stimulates the pituitary gland to release adrenocorticotrophic hormone, which in turn stimulates the adrenal glands to release the stress hormone cortisol. Cortisol is known to play an important role in the development of metabolic syndrome, major depression, and Alzheimer's dementia.

It is not yet clear if rhodiola is of significant benefit in preventing or alleviating the symptoms and pathology of Alzheimer's or other forms of dementia. However, the herb has promise, and it appears to be a benign substance with few if any adverse effects. There have been cautionary notes that people diagnosed with bipolar affective disorder should not take preparations of rhodiola without supervision from a physician.

S-ADENOSYLMETHIONINE (SAMe)

S-adenosylmethionine (SAMe) is an ancient and important substance in biology. It is necessary for normal function in both plants and animals.

It is found in every cell in the human body and in organisms as primitive as *E. coli* bacteria. SAMe is the primary donor of single carbon atoms, or methyl groups. Dozens of critical biochemical interactions depend upon the transfer of a methyl group from one molecule to another. The vitamins folate and B_1 perform most of their essential work by transferring methyl groups. SAMe also plays a role in the synthesis of a number of important neurotransmitters, which is part of the reason that it has been found to be helpful in the treatment of major depression. SAMe is the methyl donor in the synthesis of the choline component of the neurotransmitter acetylcholine and in the methylation of N-acetyl-5-hydroxytryptamine, which generates melatonin in the body. A major means by which DNA is activated or deactivated is methylation of specific sites on the DNA molecule.

The healthy human body almost certainly produces sufficient amounts of SAMe. However, there is evidence that supplementation with SAMe may improve a number of conditions that might otherwise increase the risk of dementia. SAMe reduces insulin resistance when given to OLETF rats, which is a strain of rat that tends to develop diabetes type 2. SAMe can reverse some of the adverse effects of metabolic syndrome on liver function. Liver function in individuals with the so-called fatty liver of metabolic syndrome is improved by SAMe. SAMe improves liver function in alcoholic liver disease. SAMe also reduces blood levels of the inflammatory signal TNF, which are elevated in metabolic syndrome.

It has recently been suggested that deficiency of SAMe may contribute to the development of Alzheimer's disease. Studies have shown that SAMe levels are low in cerebrospinal fluid and brain tissue of patients with Alzheimer's disease. SAMe levels are reduced by up to 85 percent in some areas of these patients' brains. However, several other studies have revealed no differences between healthy and demented individuals in their brain levels of SAMe. There are a number of ways by which inadequate levels of SAMe could increase the risk of dementia. Because SAMe contributes methyl groups for the synthesis of choline, deficiency of SAMe may lead to the diminished levels of acetylcholine that characterize Alzheimer's dementia. SAMe also plays an important role in the control of gene expression in the brain by adding methyl groups to certain sections of DNA and thus turning them off. SAMe methylates two genes responsible for controlling expression of amyloid protein. Decreases in SAMe-mediated methylation of the presenilin 1 and beta-secretase genes allows overexpression of "sticky" forms of amyloid that accumulate as plaques in Alzheimer's dementia. In human cell cultures, addition of SAMe reduces amyloid production. Other data suggests that increases in S-adenosylhomocysteine, a metabolite of SAMe that accumulates in the absence of sufficient folate, B_{12}, and SAMe, prevents the usual ability of cells to rid themselves of hyperphosphorylated tau. Hyperphosphorylated tau protein is what forms the neurofibrillary tangles of Alzheimer's dementia.

SAMe restored working memory function in rats whose brains had been damaged by transient loss of blood supply. In a French study, old dogs that displayed evidence of what was described as "age-related mental impairment" were given SAMe for two months. Mental impairment was improved by 50 percent in many of those animals. Unfortunately, the only published trial of using SAMe to treat active Alzheimer's dementia showed a lack of efficacy. It is tempting to speculate that earlier intervention may have been more successful.

It is commonly believed that simply increasing intake of folate and vitamin B_{12} provides many of the same benefits as supplementing with SAMe. In most individuals, this is probably the case. However, some individuals, including many who have had difficult-to-treat major depression, may have systems that do not properly process folate. Such people often have an aberrant form of an important enzyme called methylenetetrahydrofolate reductase, or MTHFR. One particular form of MTHFR of concern is referred to as MTHFR C677T, and the presence of this variant is thought to result in inadequate synthesis of SAMe in the body and brain. Although it remains controversial, there is existing data suggesting that individuals with the MTHFR C677T gene are at increased risk for dementia. It is now possible to test for the presence of aberrant forms of this enzyme. SAMe can be helpful in some individuals with treatment-resistant depression who are likely to suffer this problem, and the same individuals are also likely to reduce their risk of dementia by taking SAMe. In some patients with liver disease in whom the biochemical activities of the liver, including the replenishment of SAMe by folate and B_{12}, are impaired, adding SAMe can improve liver function. There is evidence that age-related decline in liver function can also be improved with SAMe. People with this difficulty might also reduce their risk of dementia by supplementing with SAMe. For most people, the benefits of this expensive supplement are not likely to be worthwhile. The most reasonable approach is to first make certain that folate and B_{12} intake is adequate and that serum levels of homocysteine, a by-product of methionine metabolism, are normal.

SAGE

In an old Anglo-Saxon manuscript from the Middle Ages it was written, "Why should a man die if he has sage?" The sixteenth-century English physician and herbalist John Gerard said of sage, "It is singularly good for the head and brain and quickeneth the nerves and memory." Sage has been used for centuries to treat problems of memory. It was used by the ancient Egyptians and has been a staple in Chinese and Indian Ayurvedic medicines. There is now strong scientific data to support the observations of the ancients that sage can be useful for the prevention and treatment of dementia.

Sage is a plant of the genus *Salvia*, which is derived from Latin for "save" and harkens back to its use as a salve for healing. There are hundreds of species in the genus *Salvia*, and many have been used for medicinal purposes. However, there are differences among them. Some have toxic components. Diviner's sage, or *Salvia divinorum*, is hallucinogenic. Many species of sage, including *Salvia officinalis*, or simple garden sage, contain significant amounts of the substance thujone. *Salvia lavandulaefolia*, or Spanish sage, appears to have less thujone. Some may recognize that thujone is found in absinthe and may contribute to the heady and toxic effects of that infamous European drink. Modest amounts of extracts of both garden sage and Spanish sage have been used in human studies of cognitive function.

As is always the case with herbs, sage is complex and contains a variety of active substances. One of the main active ingredients is likely to be rosmarinic acid, which, not surprisingly, is also found in the common garden herb rosemary. Sage also contains cineole, pinene, borneol, carophylene, linalool, and other substances. Camphor contributes to the strong fragrance of many types of sages. More than one of these substances are likely to contribute to the benefits of sage.

Standard neuropharmacological tests have demonstrated that components of sage can increase activity of acetylcholine in the brain by inhibiting the actions of the enzymes acetylcholinesterase and butyrylcholinesterase. This is the same mechanism of action of most of the medications prescribed for Alzheimer's dementia. Of particular interest are studies showing that the rosmarinic acid in sage protects the brain from many of the toxic effects of amyloid protein, including stimulation of hyperphosphorylation of tau, which is responsible for neurofibrillary tangles. In addition, certain components of sage have antioxidant, anti-inflammatory, estrogenic, and sedative effects. In a recent report in the *British Journal of Nutrition*, sage oil was described as having effects similar to those of metformin, a drug often prescribed by doctors to treat diabetes type 2. Sage increases sensitivity to insulin and helps normalize blood glucose levels.

Well-performed scientific studies have begun to show that sage can favorably affect cognitive function. Single doses rapidly improve memory, attention, and mood, not only in normal adults over sixty-five, but also in healthy young adults. Initial studies also suggest that six weeks of treatment with sage oil may even improve memory and attention in patients already diagnosed with Alzheimer's dementia.

Sage appears to be a rather benign treatment. In the six-week study that primarily evaluated the safety of chronic administration of Spanish sage oil in elderly subjects with Alzheimer's dementia, no ill effects were found. This is despite the fact that this group tends to have many medical problems and physical frailties.

SOY

There would seem to be few foods as benign as the soy bean product tofu. It is touted as a health food, and it is an excellent source of cholesterol-free protein for vegetarians. Its blandness is almost the stuff of legend. Thus, it may come as a surprise that there is considerable controversy over whether it prevents or contributes to dementia. There are many studies, albeit primarily in animals, that would suggest that tofu and other soy products, including soy milk, have effects that would help protect the brain and prevent dementia. These beneficial effects have been reflected in a number of studies that have shown that soy products can improve cognitive function in people, particularly in postmenopausal women. However, there have also been several studies of human subjects showing that frequent consumption of tofu in midlife and old age can cause brain atrophy, worsening of memory, and an overall increased likelihood of dementia.

Soy beans are a staple in the Asian diet. They are an excellent source of protein. Soy products, such as whole beans, bean sprouts, tofu, and soy milk, also contain a class of compounds called isoflavones. Soy is only one of many plants that produce isoflavones; however, soy is often the primary source of isoflavones in the human diet. Isoflavones have a number of important properties that can affect human health, including brain and cognitive function. Two of the most important isoflavones in soy are genistein and daidzein. Both of these substances are potent antioxidants, which would be expected to help reduce oxidative stress, inflammation, and other sources of damage in the brain and other tissues. In old female rats, soy isoflavones increase the production of BDNF, which stimulates growth of neurons and is thought to help protect against dementia and major depression. In an impressive study of female monkeys made "postmenopausal" by surgical removal of their ovaries, soy isoflavones were found to reduce the hyperphosphorylation of tau protein in their brains. Hyperphosphorylated tau is the abnormal substance that forms neurofibrillary tangles in the brains of patients with Alzheimer's dementia. Genistein also appears to reduce the neurotoxic effects of beta amyloid protein in the brains of rodents.

Several studies have shown that postmenopausal women treated with isoflavones extracted from soy have improved cognitive function, including improved verbal fluency and memory. Another study showed improvements in planning and mental flexibility, both of which are functions of the frontal lobes of the brain, but no improvement in memory. As if the beneficial effects of soy on the brain and cognitive function I have noted weren't enough, both of the major isoflavones found in soy also have significant ability to block the beginning of cancerous growth of cells. In fact, several large epidemiological studies have suggested that the high intake of soy products by Japanese women is at least partially responsible for their lower risk of developing breast cancer than American women. There is even some indication that the genistein in soy may help prevent prostate cancer. Addition of soy to the diet improves features of the metabolic syndrome in animals and humans. This includes increases in insulin sensitivity and improvement in blood glucose, cholesterol, and triglyceride levels. So far, soy sounds as if it were a miracle cure-all.

The study that has caused so much concern and confusion about soy is one that was performed as part of the large and well-regarded Honolulu-Asia Aging Study. In this study it was found that men who in their forties and fifties ate two or more servings of tofu a week had an increased likelihood of brain atrophy and poor cognitive performance when tested roughly thirty years later. A similar finding was produced in a very recent study of men and women in Indonesia in which high intake of tofu was again associated with poor memory. This study, which was funded by the British Alzheimer's Research Trust and performed by experienced university researchers, must also be seen as significant and concerning. What in the world does all of this mean?

Some of the ability of isoflavones to reduce the risk of breast and prostate cancer may arise from the fact that these substances also have effects at estrogen receptors in the human body. In fact, many of the isoflavones are in a class of compounds called phytoestrogens, which simply means "estrogens from plant sources." As I noted in an earlier chapter, the effects of estrogens on the brain, and their ability to cause or prevent dementia, has become confusing and controversial. I suspect that the confusion over the effects of soy, with its phytoestrogens, on dementia is very similar to that seen in studies of estrogens and estrogen replacement therapy and dementia. The effects of soy and the phytoestrogens it contains on dementia and health in general remain important areas of research by doctors, nutritionists, and neuroscientists. Hopefully, we can expect some clarification of these questions over the next five to ten years.

For those of you who absolutely love tofu (and I am talking to *both* of you), there is not enough solid information to tell you to stop. This is particularly true if you are a woman and a vegetarian who depends on soy as a good source of protein. However, if you are able to reduce your consumption of tofu or soy milk to fewer than two servings a week, it would be a prudent step to take. If you are male, I would avoid consuming tofu or soy milk more than once or twice a month.

VINPOCETINE

Vinpocetine is a synthetic chemical that is made by slightly altering the natural substance vincamine, which is extracted from the leaf of the lesser periwinkle plant. Vinpocetine has been given the trade name Cavinton, and it has been sold in Eastern Europe and Japan since the late 1970s as a treatment for decline in cognitive function. In the United States it has been available over the counter in health food stores and on the Internet.

Vinpocetine has been studied and its effects described in well-regarded scientific journals. There is scientific basis to conclude that vinpocetine might very well be of value in preventing or reversing certain types of cognitive decline. Vinpocetine has antioxidant effects that can protect the brain from oxidative stress, which is increased in metabolic syndrome, diabetes, and inflammatory states. Vinpocetine has been found to reduce some of the damage caused by exposure of the brain to amyloid. It appears to be particularly helpful in protecting mitochondria from effects of amyloid that are believed to be due to increases in oxidative stress. Vinpocetine can also act to reduce activity at specific sodium channels in neurons in the brain. Blocking these sodium channels slows activity of the neurons and is thought to offer some protection against what is referred to as "excitotoxicity," which results from neurons being overstimulated. This type of excitotoxicity can occur after a stroke or even on an ongoing basis in brain tissue of patients with various forms of dementia.

Indications are that vinpocetine is probably most useful in treating the cognitive decline that occurs in the early stages of vascular dementia. Vinpocetine is known to act as an inhibitor of the enzyme phosphodiesterase type 1 (PDE-1). This enzyme is found in the inner lining of blood vessels. Blocking PDE-1 activity leads to relaxation of the blood vessel, which in turn leads to improvement in blood flow. Ultrasound measurements of blood flow in the brain have shown that twelve weeks of treatment with vin-pocetine increases blood flow in arteries that supply the brain. In patients who had previously suffered strokes or shown other signs of having vascular insufficiency, twelve weeks of vinpocetine improved cognitive function. Among these patients were some who were merely suffering MCI and had not progressed to diagnoses of dementia.

Both clinical studies and knowledge of the mechanism of action of vin-pocetine suggest that it may be of value in treating patients with vascular insufficiency who suffer either MCI or actual vascular dementia. Unfortunately, there is little if any evidence that it is useful in treating or preventing Alzheimer's dementia. One of the first evaluations of vinpocetine, performed at a Veterans Administration hospital in 1989, found that while vinpocetine had no significant adverse effects, it neither improved nor delayed the progressive loss of cognitive function in patients with Alzheimer's dementia. In 2003, the Cochrane reviewers reported that their review of the literature revealed no indications that vinpocetine was useful in the prevention or treatment of dementia. It is important to note, however, that they clearly stated that it in most studies it was not possible to determine if subjects suffered Alzheimer's versus vascular dementia. Thus, it is possible that benefits of vinpocetine treatment for vascular dementia may have been masked by lack of benefit in patients with Alzheimer's dementia.

As I have mentioned before, it may be difficult to differentiate vascular dementia from Alzheimer's or other forms of dementia. Moreover, "pure" vascular or Alzheimer's dementias are more likely the exception rather than the rule, as most sufferers show signs of "mixed" dementias. This is important and something you should discuss with your doctor. Existing high blood pressure, history of strokes or transient ischemic attacks (sometimes called reversible or "pre-" strokes), angina, history of heart attacks, intermittent claudication, or your doctor's confirmation of atherosclerosis may warrant suspicion of vascular insufficiency. If this is the case, there may be some value in taking vinpocetine. In studies in which vinpocetine was found to be both safe and effective for treatment of vascular dementia, doses of 10 mg were taken three times a day.

VITAMIN A

Increasing evidence is showing that vitamin A deficiency may contribute to the development of several different types of dementia, including Alzheimer's and Lewy body dementias. Unfortunately, whereas taking too much of most vitamins causes little more than expensive urine, taking too much vitamin A can cause serious harm. Thus, great care must be taken in supplementing the diet with any of the various forms of vitamin A.

Vitamin A is a family of substances that are found in foods of both animal and plant origin. Animals of all species store most of the vitamin A they consume in their livers. Cod liver oil, of which so many older individuals have such fond memories, is an excellent source of the vitamin. Beef or chicken liver are also good sources. Likely the best source of vitamin A is the liver of the polar bear. In fact, polar bear liver is so rich in vitamin A that a single serving can be lethal. There have been reports of arctic explorers dying from hypervitaminosis A after eating the livers of polar bears. Vitamin A from animal sources is in the form of retinol. Variations of animal-derived vitamin A, such as retinyl palmitate, can also be found in some vitamin tablets. Because of its potential toxicity, care must be taken not to take too much vitamin A. Moreover, because it is stored away in the liver and soluble in fat, mildly toxic doses of vitamin A from animal sources can accumulate over time with dangerous results. Plant sources of vitamin A are primarily green leafy vegetables and orange or yellow vegetables and fruit. The forms of vitamin A from plants, such as the beta-carotene in carrots, are considered "provitamins," and need to be converted into useable form in the body. In contrast, the retinyl palmitate and other animal sources of vitamin A are referred to as "preformed." Provitamins are far less toxic than preformed vitamin A, as there are limits to the degree that they can be converted to retinol and other active forms.

Vitamin A is best known for its role in vision. The term "retinol" comes from the fact that the retina of the eye contains a great deal of vitamin A. The retina uses this indispensable substance in converting light into a chemical signal that can be appreciated by the nervous system. Vitamin A in the form of retinoic acid is needed for normal growth and maintenance of skin cells, as well as cells that line important organs, such as the lungs and digestive tract. The vitamin also plays an important role in immune function and bone maintenance.

Vitamin A deficiency is relatively rare in developed countries. Moreover, it is seen more often in children than adults. Nonetheless, poor diet or digestive problems can result in deficiencies. Because of its importance in vision, one of the first manifestations of vitamin A deficiency is "night blindness." Rough, dry skin is another symptom of vitamin A deficiency. It has recently been found that lack of vitamin A can increase the risk of dementia.

Test tube studies have shown that retinol, retinoic acid, and beta-carotene can all prevent the crystallization of alpha-synuclein protein, which is the abnormal process seen in Lewy body dementia. Similar studies have shown these forms of vitamin A to reduce formation of beta amyloid. A year with deficient vitamin A in the diet increases deposition of amyloid protein in the brain tissue of rats, whereas replacement of vitamin A helps reverse this abnormality. There is also evidence that vitamin A is necessary for proper function of the hippocampus, which is an area that sustains severe damage in dementia. Low, but not high, doses of retinoic acids stimulate neurogenesis in the hippocampus of the mouse. Studies using mice have also found that decreases in activation of vitamin A receptors in the brain parallel age-related losses in memory and learning. Supplementing these animals with vitamin A throughout their lives counteracts those age-related losses in cognitive function. Along with these direct effects on the brain, vitamin A is also known to improve insulin resistance and reduce inflammatory activity by blocking effects of the inflammation trigger NF-κB. These effects would also help to dampen neurodegenerative processes.

In most, though not all, studies, blood levels of vitamin A are lower in patients with Alzheimer's dementia than in normal, age-matched subjects. Moreover, vitamin A levels are known to decrease in the brain with age, with this decrease tending to be more marked in the brains of patients with Alzheimer's dementia. All together, these findings would suggest that a lack of vitamin A might contribute to the development of dementia, particularly Alzheimer's and Lewy body dementias. Unfortunately, there have not been any large or definitive studies to determine what if any effects vitamin A supplementation has on the prevention or alleviation of dementia in human subjects.

Because the types of vitamin A can be so different, doses of the vitamin are standardized as retinol activity equivalents, or RAEs. An RAE is a microgram of retinol or 2 mcg of beta-carotene. Another way to express this is in International Units, or IUs. An RAE is equivalent to 3.3 IUs of vitamin A. The current recommended daily allowance (RDA) of vitamin A for men is 900 RAEs, which is 900 mcg of retinol, 1800 mcg of beta-carotene, or any form of vitamin A standardized as 3,000 IUs. For women, the RDA is 700 RAEs, 700 mcg of retinol, 1400 mcg of beta-carotene, or about 2,300 IU.

As I have noted, high intake of preformed vitamin A can be dangerous or even lethal. Hair loss, poor coordination, headache, bone and muscle pain, and, most seriously, liver damage can result from hypervitaminosis A. Chronic intake of doses of vitamin A only twice the RDA have been reported to increase osteoporosis and contribute to bone fractures. Women of childbearing age must be particularly vigilant against overindulgence in vitamin A, as high doses can cause birth defects. Daily doses of 10,000 IU a day, about four times the RDA, are known to be sufficient to cause such defects. Because deficiency is relatively rare and too high an intake of vita-min A can be toxic, it is unwise to take anything more than the RDA of vi-tamin A. Because it is far less toxic and a better antioxidant than preformed vitamin A, it may be wiser to take the provitamin form of beta-carotene. Thus, I recommend a daily dose of 1400 mcg beta-carotene for women and 1800 mcg for men. Along with a healthy and varied diet, this will give you a healthy supply of a safe form of vitamin A.

VITAMIN C

In past centuries, sailors who voyaged on long journeys across the seas were prone to developing a constellation of symptoms that included bruising of the skin, fragile bones, bleeding, loss of teeth, and weakness. The condition was called scurvy. A Scottish naval surgeon named James Lind discovered that the addition of lime juice to the diets of British sailors prevented them from developing the dreaded and sometimes fatal disease. Nonetheless, scurvy had killed tens of thousands of sailors from all nations, and it con-tinued to do so for years even after Lind's first publication of his results in 1753. It wasn't until 1928 that the "ascorbic," or scurvy-preventing sub-stance, in lime juice and other fruits and vegetables was actually isolated and identified. This was done at virtually the same time independently by two different groups of researchers led by Albert Szent-Gyorgyi and Charles G. King.

Ascorbic acid is often referred to as vitamin C. Most mammals are able to synthesize vitamin C in their bodies, and they do not suffer scurvy-like symptoms if their diets are deficient in the vitamin. However, through evo-lution, humans, other primates, fruit bats, and the humble guinea pig have all lost the capacity to synthesize vitamin C. We depend on our diets to provide enough vitamin C to remain healthy. Although vitamin C is clearly established to be an essential nutrient in the diet, there continues to be controversy over how much vitamin C is necessary, and if the RDA is the same as the amount we need for optimal health. Currently, the National Academy of Sciences' RDA for vitamin C is 75 mg a day for women and 90 mg a day for men. Smokers are advised to take an additional 35 mg a day.

Most people are aware of the controversy that arose when Dr. Linus Paul-ing recommended that adults take 10 grams of vitamin C each day, which was nearly twenty times larger than the RDA. Pauling himself took 18 grams of vitamin C daily. Please let me emphasize that Linus Pauling, winner of Nobel Prizes for chemistry and peace, was no fool! He possessed, and put to great use, one of the best minds of the twentieth century. Pauling did not come up with his figure of 10 grams per day by mere speculation. He derived this amount by calculating how much vitamin C is made each day in the bodies of animals that retained the biochemical machinery to synthesize the substance, and then extrapolating to human beings. It is quite possible, however, that Pauling did not take into account the likelihood that humans, who do not make our own vitamin C, may also have evolved to possess an ability to need less than one might expect from comparisons to other animals. This appears to be the case, and the Linus Pauling Institute, which is now situated on the campus of Oregon State University, has modified Pauling's original recommendation to suggest that healthy, non-smoking adults take 400 mg of vitamin C per day.

Vitamin C plays many important roles in the body. The bruising, fragile bones, and tooth loss in scurvy were due to the fact that vitamin C is necessary to produce the structural protein collagen. Vitamin C is also necessary for the synthesis of the neurotransmitters serotonin, norepinephrine, and epinephrine. One of the most important roles that vitamin C plays is as an antioxidant. Vitamin C has been found to reduce the toxicity of amyloid in brain tissue by blocking amyloid-induced influxes of calcium into neurons in the brain. This is thought to be due to antioxidant effects of vitamin C. Enzymes in the brain that break down amyloid can suffer oxidative damage and lose the ability to rid the brain of the abnormal protein. Vitamin C helps maintain the activity of these enzymes.

A number of studies have shown that people with Alzheimer's dementia tend to have low levels of vitamin C and other antioxidants in their blood. This has also been seen in people diagnosed as having MCI. These deficiencies may be due in part to lower intake of vitamin C. However, it has also been found that patients with Alzheimer's tend to have lower blood levels of vitamin C even when dietary intake of the vitamin is normal. This may be due to the fact that people with Alzheimer's dementia have a high ongoing level of oxidative stress, and vitamin C gets used up more rapidly than it does in people without the illness.

Because oxidative stress is responsible for so much of the damage caused by metabolic syndrome and is an important trigger of inflammation and damage in neurodegenerative diseases, it is reasonable to suspect that a deficiency of vitamin C would increase the risk of developing dementia. Conversely, one might further suspect that increasing the intake of vitamin C would provide extra protection against dementia. Unfortunately, results of studies of the ability of vitamin C supplementation to prevent or treat dementia have been inconsistent.

One large and well-known study, the Honolulu-Asia Aging Study, found that there was no relationship between the amount of vitamin C consumed in the daily diet during midlife (ages forty-five to sixty-eight) and likelihood of developing Alzheimer's dementia over the following twenty-five years. In another large but briefer study, vitamin C was found to be an important factor in reducing the risk of dementia. There appeared to be a roughly 10 percent decrease in likelihood of dementia with each 100 mg of vitamin C consumed per day. Unfortunately, dementia was measured simply as changes in the MMSE score, and no attempt was made to determine what type of dementia might be involved. Researchers did comment, however, that the known decrease in strokes in people who take vitamin C supplements suggested that at least some of the protection from cognitive impairment was likely due to decreases in the risk of vascular dementia. Overall, most studies of effects of vitamin C find no measurable benefit of the vitamin in reducing the risk of dementia. Several studies that did find reductions in the risk of dementia saw these reductions in people who took *both* vitamin C and vitamin E.

Overall, what I believe can be stated from what we have learned from studies of vitamin C is that taking vitamin C in combination with vitamin E can help to slightly reduce the risk of Alzheimer's and vascular dementias. Vitamin C should probably be taken in the 400 mg per day dose currently suggested by the Linus Pauling Institute. There are no studies suggesting that vitamin C is able to reverse or slow the progression of a diagnosed case of Alzheimer's or other form of dementia.

VITAMIN D

Vitamin D is generally thought of as "the sunshine vitamin," necessary for the development and maintenance of strong bones. The best-known effects of vitamin D are the enhancement of absorption of calcium from the gut and control of the deposition of minerals in the bones. The lack of vitamin D in growing children causes the now rare bone condition called rickets. Vitamin D deficiency can also contribute to osteoporosis, that is, weak, porous bones, in adults. However, the variety and importance of vitamin D's activities in the body are far greater than even most physicians have ever realized. Vitamin D affects calcium metabolism not only in the bones, but in the brain as well. There it affects the production of nerve growth factors and neurotransmitters. It helps control cell growth, differentiation, and apoptosis of various cell types in the brain and other organs in the body.

It plays a role in modulating immune responses and in controlling release of insulin and the body's sensitivity to that hormone. There is growing evidence that the importance of vitamin D ranges far beyond the maintenance of strong bones and may include the prevention and treatment of metabolic syndrome, diabetes, heart disease, certain forms of cancer, major depression, and dementia.

Vitamin D deficiency can increase the risk of a number of conditions that increase the likelihood of developing dementia. Several studies have shown that vitamin D deficiency increases insulin resistance and the risk of developing metabolic syndrome. Insufficient vitamin D results in poor glucose tolerance, hypertension, and increased risk of diabetes type 2. Vitamin D is known to blunt the inflammatory response, and it has been shown to lower concentrations of markers of inflammation in the blood of people diagnosed with metabolic syndrome. Lack of vitamin D may thus allow inflammatory processes to spin out of control. This is why vitamin D deficiency is associated with the inflammatory illness rheumatoid arthritis, as well as with the bone weakness disease osteoporosis. Vitamin D deficiency adversely affects blood lipids and exacerbates high blood pressure. In the large United States government–sponsored Third National Health and Nutrition Examination Survey, vitamin D deficiency was found to be an independent risk factor for the development of cardiovascular disease.

Vitamin D receptors are found throughout the brain, including in the limbic system, which is involved in the processing of emotion. There is growing evidence that vitamin D deficiency plays a role in the development of major depression and the wintertime blues illness known as seasonal affective disorder. Density of vitamin D receptors is particularly high in the hippocampus, which is involved in learning and memory. Several studies have shown a direct relationship between the level of vitamin D in the blood and cognitive performance on the Mini-Mental State Examination. In one study of patients already diagnosed with Alzheimer's dementia, higher vitamin D levels were also associated with higher cognitive function scores. Surprisingly, those higher scores were more strongly correlated with vitamin D levels than with those of vitamins B_1, B_6, and B_{12}, which are more often associated with cognitive function.

Many sufferers of Alzheimer's disease are deficient in vitamin D, and their brains have relatively low numbers of vitamin D receptors. Certain abnormal subtypes of vitamin receptors in the brain have also recently been associated with increased risk for developing Alzheimer's dementia. Low vitamin D levels are similarly seen in Parkinson's disease, which is closely related to Lewy body dementia.

There are many means by which adequate vitamin D levels could help protect the brain from neurodegenerative disease. It stimulates production of neural growth factors that maintain the health of neurons in the brain. It stimulates production of the brain proteins calmodulin and calbindin, which mediate neurogenesis and other critical functions. The antioxidant effects of vitamin D are known to protect the brain from oxidative damage. Vitamin D helps protect the brain against the damage caused by chronic high levels of stress hormones. In rat brains, pretreatment with vitamin D prevents the shrinkage and deaths of hippocampal neurons that occurs with exposure to the drug dexamethasone, a drug that mimics many of the effects of the stress hormone cortisol. Other studies using rats have found that vitamin D helps maintain the production of the neurotransmitter acetylcholine in specific areas of the brain. Although the use of vitamin D to decrease the risk of dementia might seem promising, to the best of my knowledge no scientific studies have been performed to determine whether supplementing with vitamin D can prevent or improve symptoms of any form of dementia.

There are two natural sources of vitamin D, sunlight and diet. The human body is perfectly capable of synthesizing 100 percent of the vitamin D it needs by exposure of the skin to sunlight. However, many people do not get sufficient exposure to sunlight. Exposure to sunlight varies considerably as the seasons change. People expose less skin when covering up against exposure to the cold of winter. Decrease in day length during the winter and the sun tracking low in the sky also diminishes the amount of sunlight that reaches the skin and thus further reduces the rate of synthesis of vitamin D. Spring and summer are the seasons of sunlight; however, legitimate concerns about skin cancer have led to widespread use of sunscreen lotions. Most sunscreens block the ultraviolet rays that generate vitamin D in the skin. Even a relatively weak SPF 8 lotion applied to the skin can almost completely eliminate the synthesis of vitamin D.

Obtaining vitamin D from the diet can bypass the problem of low exposure to sunlight. Unfortunately, many adults do not consume sufficient amounts of vitamin D–containing food products, such as fortified milk. Consequently, vitamin D deficiency is far more prevalent than many physicians suspect. In a study of healthy, young hospital workers in Boston, 36 percent of them were deficient in vitamin D by the end of the winter. A recent review reveals that as many as 57 percent of general medicine inpatients in the United States suffer from inadequate levels of vitamin D.

The solution to vitamin D deficiency by supplementation is simple. A healthy individual need only take 10 to 20 micrograms, or 400 to 800 IU of vitamin D daily to prevent deficiency. Because vitamin D can be toxic in high quantities, there is no compelling reason to take more than 800 IU a day.

VITAMIN E

Vitamin E is a family of related substances that are required by the body to remain healthy. The E vitamins are divided into two main groups, the tocopherols and the tocotriens. These main groups themselves also consist of subtypes. Alpha-tocopherol is most plentiful in the human body, and it is the form most often found in vitamin E supplements. Gamma-tocopherol is probably the next most important subtype of vitamin E, and it is quite common in nuts, seeds, and vegetable oils, particularly the corn and soy bean oils that are increasingly common in the modern diet.

Doses of vitamin E are usually measured as IU, rather than milligrams. This can be confusing. The IU is used because while the various members of the "vitamin E family" do much the same thing in the body, they differ from one another in their potency per milligram in doing so. Thus, to insure a necessary amount of vitamin E activity, rather than a number of milligrams that might not be sufficiently effective, vitamin E is standardized in units based on the activity of a specific amount of alpha-tocopherol. The FDA's recommended daily allowance of vitamin E is 15 IU for an adult. The best natural sources of vitamin E in the diet are vegetable oils, nuts, seeds, and green leafy vegetables.

The E vitamins are fat soluble, and their main function is to protect the body from substances that can oxidize and damage fatty molecules in the membranes that enclose every cell. Brain cells, with their high level of oxygen usage, are particularly prone to oxidative damage and are thus in need of extra protection. When oxidation by dangerous substances called free radicals begins, a chain of damaging oxidation reactions can occur, with not only fat, but protein, DNA, and other important molecules at risk for attack.

LDL cholesterol is yet another fatty substance vulnerable to oxidation. Oxidized LDL plays a major role in the initiation and progression of atherosclerosis in small arteries of the heart, brain, and other organs. Reduction in the rate of LDL oxidation is possibly what makes supplementation with vitamin E effective in reducing the risk of coronary artery disease. There is some evidence that vitamin E may also help reduce serum cholesterol and protect the body from certain cancers. However, those possible benefits of vitamin E are less well established. In rat brains, vitamin E has been found to enhance the process of neurogenesis and decrease rates of neuron death.

In mouse models of Alzheimer's dementia, lack of vitamin E increases deposition of beta amyloid in brain tissue.

A number of studies have been performed to evaluate the use of vitamin E in treating Alzheimer's dementia in humans. Unfortunately, vitamin E offers few if any benefits to patients who have already been diagnosed as having the illness. On the other hand, several reports, including a large 2004 study performed at Johns Hopkins University, suggest that vitamin E may help prevent the initial development of Alzheimer's dementia. In that study, vitamin E was found to be effective only when taken along with vitamin C. These two antioxidants are known to work together to bolster each other's effects.

In view of vitamin E's ability to decrease oxidation of LDL and reduce the risk of cardiovascular disease, it seems reasonable to suspect that it might also reduce the risk of developing vascular dementia. At least one group found that diets rich in vitamin E do tend to reduce the risk of vascular dementia. Conversely, patients with vascular dementia have been found to have lower levels of vitamin E than patients with Alzheimer's dementia. Similarly, patients with the Binswanger's form of vascular dementia use up vitamin E at a rate faster than is seen in Alzheimer's patients. In some European studies, up to 25 percent of otherwise normal elderly subjects are found to have low blood levels of vitamin E. This would suggest that many people might benefit from vitamin E supplementation. Still, the majority of studies have failed to find strong evidence that increasing one's intake of vitamin E can significantly reduce the risk of developing vascular dementia. There are no studies about the use of vitamin E in treating or preventing frontotemporal or Lewy body dementia. However, there are studies showing that vitamin E can help reduce the risk of developing Parkinson's disease, which is similar in many ways to Lewy body dementia.

Vitamin E activity is standardized with the basic assumption that all forms of the vitamin, whether they are alpha or gamma, tocopherol or tocotrien, do exactly the same things in the body, only with differing potencies in doing so. However, some forms of vitamin E may have unique abilities and functions that have so far escaped our ability to discern them. There is evidence, for example, that gamma-tocopherol may have anti-inflammatory effects that alpha-tocopherol does not possess. There is also some evidence that gamma-tocopherol may be slightly more effective than alpha-tocopherol in reducing the risk of developing Alzheimer's dementia. High doses of alpha-tocopherol, the form found in most vitamin supplements, may lower the body's levels of gamma-tocopherol. All in all, it seems prudent to balance the intake of the various subtypes of vitamin E.

Table 6.1. Anti-Dementia Effects of Vitamins, Herbs, and Nutraceuticals

	Antioxidant	Anti-Inflammatory	Neuron Growth Stimulator	Anti-Amyloid	Acetylcholine Enhancer	Anti-Metabolic Syndrome
Acetyl-Carnitine	++	++	++	0	++	++
Alpha-Lipoic Acid	++++	+++	0	0	++	+++
Ashwagandha	+	+++	++	0	+++	++
Camosine	++	0	0	0	0	0
Chocolate	+++	++	0	0	0	++
Chromium	0	0	0	0	0	++++
Co-Enzyme Q10	+	0	0	0	0	+
Coffee	++	++	++	++	0	+
Curcumin	++	++	0	++	0	++
CDP-Choline	0	+	++	++	+++	0
DHEA	0	++	++	0	+	++
Fish Oil	0	++	++	++	0	++
Garlic	++	++	0	+	0	++
Ginkgo	++	+	++	++	+	0
Ginseng	++	++	++	0	+	++
GPC	0	0	0	0	+++	0
Grape Seed Extract	+++	+++	0	0	0	++

Green Tea	+++	++	0	++	++	++
Huperzine	++	+	++	++	++++	0
Ibuprofen	+	++++	0	++	0	++
Idebenone	+++	++	++	0	0	0
Lemon Balm	++	0	0	0	++	0
Melatonin	+++	+++	+++	++	++	++
Phosphatidylserine	+	++	++	0	+++	0
Red Yeast Rice	+	+	0	++	0	++
Resveratrol	++	++	0	++	0	++
Rhodiola	++	0	0	0	++	0
SAMe	++	+	0	++	+	0
Sage	++	+	++	0	++	++
Soy	++	++	0	0	0	++
Vinpocetine	++	0	++	0	0	0
Vitamin A	++++	++	0	++	0	++
Vitamin C	++++	0	0	0	0	0
Vitamin D	+	++	0	0	0	+
Vitamin E	++++	++	++	++	0	0

Notes: 0 = no effect; + = possible effect; ++ = mild effect; +++ = moderate effect; ++++ = strong effect.

It is imperative to note recent reports that in people over the age of sixty, high doses of vitamin E, some as high as 2000 IU a day, increase the risk of untimely death by as much as 10 percent. These findings may reflect the fact that many of these individuals were taking synthetic preparations of vitamin E that are 50/50 combinations of natural D-alpha-tocopherol and unnatural L-alpha-tocopherol. Nonetheless, until the exact cause of this apparent toxic effect of vitamin E supplementation is learned, there are prudent steps to take. One is to maximize the intake of vitamin E from food, such as whole grains, vegetable oils, and green leafy vegetables. The other is to find supplements of vitamin E from natural sources that contain a mixture of tocopherols and limit intake to no more than 400 IU a day.

7

HOW TO AVOID DEMENTIA

In 1994, Dr. K. Warner Schaie, who led the Seattle Longitudinal Study of normal aging and cognitive function, wrote a paper for the journal *American Psychologist*. In that paper he described his studies of successful aging over the previous thirty-five years. He concluded by listing what he believed to be the major factors that allowed men and women to avoid dementia and maintain healthy cognitive function throughout their lives and into old age.

Schaie noted that good health, with an absence of cardiovascular disease and other chronic illnesses, was a major factor in maintaining normal cognitive function. We know now that one of the most important conditions to avoid is metabolic syndrome and the abnormalities associated with it, which include high blood glucose, abdominal obesity, high levels of triglycerides and bad cholesterol, low levels of good cholesterol, and high blood pressure. Metabolic syndrome not only contributes to cardiovascular disease, but also to diabetes, depression, sleep apnea, and a panoply of other pathological conditions that cause or contribute to dementia. Good nutrition, exercise, restful sleep, and stress reduction are the major means by which these conditions can be avoided or, at least, controlled.

Schaie recognized the simple logic of "use it or lose it" as a strategy to maintain good cognitive function. In a 1997 interview, he said, "If you don't exercise your muscles, they get flabby. If your brain isn't stimulated, you don't keep growing the new connections that are necessary to maintain optimal mental functioning. The worst thing people do to themselves, particularly when they retire, is they say: 'Oh, I've worked all my life, now I deserve to do nothing.'" He summed it up by saying, "If you don't do anything, pretty soon you can't do anything."

We have learned in scientific studies that individuals with good educations and interesting, challenging jobs tend to avoid dementia as they age. People who stay active, read, enjoy the arts, pursue creative hobbies, travel, and continue their educations have a good chance of maintaining good cognitive function. Even people who have already been diagnosed with mild cognitive impairment, Alzheimer's, or other forms of dementia can improve their cognitive function and slow the rate of its decline by engaging in stimulating mental activities.

Schaie included being married to a spouse with high cognitive function as a helpful factor in maintaining cognitive function. He also noted the importance of keeping company with active, interesting people who provide stimulation and fresh ideas. There is increasing scientific evidence that we must also nourish and exercise the social, emotional, and spiritual aspects of ourselves to maintain our mental vitality. As social creatures, we need the love and companionship of others to fully exercise our humanity and to complete our role in the cycle of life. Finding joy in other people is an important part of enjoying life and staying active, motivated, and rewarded.

Schaie understood that feeling satisfied with one's life and accomplishments by midlife were factors associated with healthy cognitive function in old age. On the other hand, bitterness, remorse, and dissatisfaction were seen as a road to withdrawal, despair, and deterioration. We now know that depression, anxiety, and stress are major contributors to the degenerative processes that lead to dementia, and these contributions are as palpable and physical as high blood pressure, stroke, or heart attacks. In some cases, mood disorders require treatment with psychotherapy or medication. However, by one means or another, finding balance, contentment, and meaning in life are necessary for successful negotiation of aging with the spirit strong and mental faculties intact.

Much has been learned in the interim about how to accomplish the tasks of successful aging described by Schaie and about the physiological mechanisms through which they help the brain resist degenerative processes that cause dementia. However, his list of factors itself remains valid and up to date. Although the pathophysiological processes that cause dementia are extraordinarily complex, the ways to avoid dementia are surprisingly simple and straightforward.

FIRST, VISIT YOUR DOCTOR

To start formulating your plan to reduce your risk of developing Alzheimer's and other dementias you must first take stock of your overall state of health. The first and most important part of this initial step is to visit your doctor and get a thorough evaluation. You need a good physical exam, including weight and blood pressure. The evaluation should also include laboratory tests for levels of LDL and HDL forms of cholesterol, triglycerides, and blood glucose to determine if you are suffering metabolic syndrome. If you have metabolic syndrome, diabetes, or cardiovascular disease, then you must have a serious discussion with your doctor as to what to do about it.

Knowledge of the degree to which you may suffer metabolic syndrome will help determine how rigorous you need to be about altering your diet and adding supplements to reduce the damage of inflammation, oxidative stress, glycation of protein, and the other adverse effects that arise with the syndrome. Obesity will require a well-planned weight-loss program, and if weight loss and improvements in diet and lifestyle don't resolve your abnormal blood pressure, cholesterol, triglycerides, and blood glucose values, then medications might be necessary. Only your doctor can prescribe such medication.

Additional blood tests such as measurement of blood C-reactive protein can help measure the level of inflammation in your body. There are also means to measure the degree of oxidation of fats in the blood and urine, which can serve as evaluations of the burden of oxidative stress in the body. Your doctor should order blood tests to evaluate your thyroid status, as well as levels of vitamins D, B_{12}, and folic acid. Homocysteine is also easily measured in the blood. An elevated homocysteine level is a risk factor for heart disease and dementia.

If your vitamin B_{12} is low, your doctor needs to find out why. Vitamin B_{12} deficiency can be due to poor diet or medications that lower the amount of the stomach acid necessary to help absorb the vitamin. However, it can also be the result of damage to the stomach lining that prevents production of a substance called "intrinsic factor," which is needed to take vitamin B_{12} across the gut into the bloodstream. This damage can often be due to infection by *Helicobacter pylori*, which is one of the bacteria suspected of being a risk factor for dementia. *Helicobacter pylori* is easily diagnosed and treated by your doctor.

If you are a woman, it is important to know how close to menopause you are, as estrogen replacement therapy is most effective when it seamlessly continues normal estrogen levels without the drops in levels that occur as the ovaries lose function at menopause. Ask your doctor about "bioidentical" replacement of your deficient hormones. If you are a man, you should be aware that testosterone levels decrease not only with age, but as yet another effect of the metabolic syndrome. Abnormally low testosterone levels can easily be corrected if diagnosed.

If you are a man or a woman and snore loudly or awaken in the morning as tired as when you went to bed, mention this to your doctor. He or she may want to perform a sleep apnea study to screen for sleep apnea.

If you have concerns about your risks for dementia, or even about what you think might be decline in your cognitive function, don't be afraid to mention this to your doctor. Some simple screening tests, such as the Mini-Mental State Examination or the Montreal Cognitive Assessment, can easily be performed in the doctor's office. Even if the results are of no concern, the score can serve as a useful baseline against which future test scores can be compared. If there is basis for concern, your doctor is the best person to pursue medical reasons for the cognitive decline, or to refer you to a psychiatrist, neurologist, or neuropsychologist for further evaluation.

Health of the brain and mind are not separate from health of the body. Health problems that were once thought to have little if any bearing on cognitive function, such as viral and bacterial infections, are coming to be seen as risk factors for dementia. The ability to fight off infections and environmental insults that could affect cognitive function as we age depend in large degree on good health maintenance.

Last but not least, if you are not up to date in your visits to your dentist, then after seeing your doctor make a dental appointment. Dental health plays a critical role in your overall health, and current evidence shows that tooth loss and gum disease are important risk factors in the development of dementia.

YOUR AGE AND YOUR PLAN TO AVOID DEMENTIA

Dementia most often begins to appear in a person's late sixties or early seventies. However, the best evidence shows that degeneration of brain tissue actually starts much earlier than that. Amyloid plaques begin to form ten years or more before any noticeable loss of memory and other signs and symptoms of dementia become apparent. Problems that contribute to amyloid deposition and neurofibrillary tangles, such as mitochondrial damage, oxidative stress, and inflammation, can begin even earlier. Metabolic syndrome, which plays such an important role in predisposing people to dementia, at first causes only subtle changes in fat, liver, and muscle cells. However, these adverse changes accumulate over many years to cause the cardiovascular disease, high blood pressure, high cholesterol, and diabetes that put people at risk for dementia. Evidence shows that the brain can also suffer damage from these conditions well before the appearance of dementia. The unfortunate fact is that even among young children, the prevalence of obesity, high blood pressure, and outright metabolic syndrome is growing at an accelerating rate. For example, the effects of poor diet and metabolic syndrome are being seen in the form of so-called fatty streaks of cholesterol deposited in the walls of the aorta and coronary arteries of the heart in children as young as their preteens. It goes without saying that among adults, these health problems are occurring in epidemic proportions. No age is too young to start living a healthy lifestyle that can reduce the risk of dementia.

For young or old, the same basic rules apply in terms of diet, stress reduction, physical exercise, attaining ideal weight, pursuing mental stimulation, enjoying good sleep, and maintaining emotional health. However, for most people under fifty who are in good health, simply making healthy lifestyle choices should be sufficient. If you are not in good health, but rather have metabolic syndrome, diabetes, heart disease, or if you have a strong family history of dementia, then even under fifty years of age, healthy lifestyle choices may not be enough. You and your doctor must address your medical conditions, you should make lifestyle changes, and it is likely time to start some of the supplements I have suggested.

There is no hard and fast rule about at what age you should start taking supplements if you are otherwise healthy and don't have a family history of dementia. It must again be noted that the degenerative changes that underlie dementia begin many years before they become obvious in one's day to day life. Thus, by the age of fifty, such supplementation is reasonable. Aside from certain caveats I have mentioned, all are safe if taken in moderation. Of course, none should be started without discussion with your doctor.

Age is clearly a factor in the decline of certain hormones and other natural substances in your body. Levels of estrogens, testosterone, melatonin, and DHEA all begin to drop as we age. Whereas replacement of these substances may be beneficial, adding such hormones when their levels are adequate is needless, expensive, and potentially dangerous. Let your physician guide you based on studies that he or she chooses out of consideration of your age. Another consideration that changes with age is the ability to tolerate exercise, as well the need for a physician's supervision in starting an exercise program.

No one is too old to benefit from a plan to improve health and lessen the risk of dementia. Even the elderly who suffer cognitive loss and have been diagnosed with MCI or dementia can benefit from exercise, mental stimulation, and relief from stress. Keep in mind that it is possible to violate rules of common sense if one is trying to manage every aspect of an elderly person's life. I recall that my own wonderful "Granny" was ninety-six years old when the staff at her nursing home told her that she couldn't have seconds on ice cream because it would raise her cholesterol. I called the nursing home and, to make a long story short, she was subsequently allowed to have seconds of ice cream whenever she wanted. Life-enhancing experiences shouldn't be dismissed out of thoughtless fear.

If you or an elderly loved one has been diagnosed with MCI or dementia, then medication in addition to the above measures is an option about which you must speak with your doctor. Many of the supplements I have described will also help and can be chosen in accordance with the effects that will complement the acetylcholine-enhancing medications that may be prescribed.

STOP METABOLIC SYNDROME, HEART DISEASE, AND DIABETES

Metabolic syndrome is occurring in epidemic proportions. Metabolic syndrome is the disease of insulin resistance, high blood pressure, high triglycerides, low HDL cholesterol, and high LDL cholesterol. Its telltale characteristic is the big belly. If metabolic syndrome persists unchecked, it propels the body toward heart disease and diabetes type 2. Those conditions are major risk factors for not only vascular dementia, but Alzheimer's and other forms of dementia as well. To reduce the risk of dementia, it is essential to control metabolic syndrome.

After your doctor has helped you determine your risk for metabolic syndrome, or perhaps the degree to which you already suffer some components of the syndrome, the rest is largely up to you. Metabolic syndrome is primarily a disease of overindulgence in carbohydrates, particularly the kinds that are rapidly digested and flood the body with sugar. Such carbohydrates are categorized as having a high glycemic index. The most obvious high glycemic index foods are pure sugar, white bread, and potato chips. However, there are many others. It is wise to purchase a glycemic index guide to help you determine which foods are least likely to stimulate unhealthy blood levels of sugar. You must also avoid the foods sweetened with high fructose corn syrup. When scientists want to produce metabolic syndrome in otherwise healthy laboratory rats for research purposes, they feed them large quantities of table sugar or fructose.

Stress stimulates the release of cortisol, which antagonizes many of the effects of insulin. Collection of fat in the abdomen disturbs the activity of fat cells and the levels of the hormones, or adipocytokines, they release. The adipocytokines, in turn, interfere with insulin sensitivity and alter the brain's control of appetite. Poor appetite control leads to more weight gain, which can lead to sleep disturbance, apnea, more stress, and more insulin resistance. The vicious, interconnected cycles quite easily spin out of control. The best way to deal with metabolic syndrome and the problems it creates, including heart disease and diabetes, is to have a healthy diet, lose weight, exercise, sleep well, and reduce stress. There are also a variety of vitamins, minerals, and nutraceuticals that can be added as supplements to help control the syndrome. If all else fails, medication may be necessary. Although medications should be used as a last resort, they shouldn't be avoided out of distaste for "artificial" means of improving your health. The fact remains that there are few medicines more dangerous than years of living with metabolic syndrome.

THE MEDITERRANEAN DIET

Diets to avoid dementia must allow people to reach and maintain their ideal weight and to minimize the major risk factors for dementia, which include metabolic syndrome, heart disease, and diabetes. The diet must also provide the brain with the unique set of nutrients it needs for nourishment, growth, and protection from the cumulative types of damage that the brain is particularly prone to, such as mitochondrial damage, oxidative stress, advanced endproduct glycation, and, of course, the deposition of amyloid plaques and neurofibrillary tangles.

The diet that for most people is the best to maintain their ideal weight and reduce the risk of metabolic syndrome and dementia is the Mediterranean diet. The Mediterranean diet is a style of eating common among the ancient cultures who have lived along the Mediterranean Coast. There is no single Mediterranean diet, rather there are many diets from those areas that share certain characteristics. A common feature among these diets is the liberal use of olive oil. The staples of these diets tend to be whole grains, beans, vegetables, fruits, and nuts. Moderate amounts of fish, poultry, and dairy products are consumed. Those dairy products are primarily yogurt and cheese, and rarely butter or cream. Only occasionally does the diet include red meat. Eggs, which are high in both cholesterol and saturated fat, are rarely eaten. Red wine is often an essential part of the meal.

The Mediterranean style of eating is characterized by low-glycemic-index carbohydrates and healthy fats. Both eliminating the type of carbohydrates that flood the body with sugar and improving the type and quantity of fat consumed in one's diet decrease the risk of developing metabolic syndrome. Consumption of large amounts of saturated fat increases insulin resistance. High intake of saturated fats also tends to result in more deposition of fat in the abdomen. Abdominal fat deposition is the pattern that predisposes one to metabolic syndrome. On the other hand, switching from saturated to mostly monounsaturated fatty acid intake, such as by replacing butter with olive oil or beef steak with salmon, increases insulin sensitivity, decreases triglycerides, and decreases LDL cholesterol. Increased intake of the omega-3 fatty acids in deep sea fish also increases insulin sensitivity and decreases triglycerides.

In Mediterranean diets, fat makes up about 30 percent of total calories, with most of the fat coming from olive oil, which is rich in monounsaturated fat. Olive oil helps improve the levels and characteristics of fat and cholesterol in the blood. The olive fruit is rich in antioxidants, so it is best to use extra virgin oil, as it retains more of these natural components. Along with olive oil, the fish, nuts, and whole grains in the Mediterranean diet provide the full range of healthy monounsaturated fats and omega-3 and omega-6 fatty acids. With low consumption of meat and dairy products, saturated fat is typically less than 10 percent of the total calories in Mediterranean diets, which meets the standards of the American Heart Association.

About 55 percent of calories in the Mediterranean diet come from carbohydrates such as whole grains, fruits, and vegetables, which are high in fiber and relatively low in glycemic index. This combination of carbohydrates improves serum glucose and increases insulin sensitivity. Pasta is also a slowly digested, low-glycemic-index source of carbohydrate, especially if served al dente and drizzled with olive oil, which slows its digestion and absorption. Thick spaghetti is preferable, as it is digested more slowly than thin pasta, such as angel hair.

Although fiber is a form of carbohydrate, it can also be seen as a distinct and important type of macronutrient. Many people think of fiber only in terms of relieving bowel irregularity. Certainly, fiber serves a very important role in this regard. However, an equally important effect of fiber is the way it changes absorption of other macronutrients. Fiber slows down the absorption of carbohydrate and acts to lower the glycemic index of high-carbohydrate foods. High fiber content in the diet lowers insulin resistance and improves serum lipids. High fiber content of food also slows the rate at which the stomach empties, and it helps give a feeling of being full. Thus, high fiber content can help reduce the number of calories consumed in each meal.

The antioxidants found in colorful fruits and vegetables, which are staples in the Mediterranean diet, have long been known to provide protection from oxidative stress and inflammation. It is no coincidence that the purples, reds, and yellows of the fruit and vegetables provide indication of their potency as antioxidants. The physics of the interaction between light and molecular structure is such that molecules with many rings of carbon, referred to as polyphenolic molecules, are deep in color as well as being best able to buffer the body against reactive oxygen radicals. Spices that give many ethnic foods their wonderful flavor and aroma, such as oregano, rosemary, and garlic, are also full of antioxidants. Red wine with meals is another common feature of the diet. Red wine contains significant amounts of antioxidants and other polyphenolic substances that reduce oxidative stress and inflammation. Modest amounts of alcohol may also help reduce the risk of heart disease and dementia.

The Mediterranean diet improves insulin sensitivity, reduces triglycerides, and improves or at least maintains HDL levels. It can prevent and even reverse metabolic syndrome, which in turn reduces the risk of heart disease. This fact is confirmed in a variety of scientific studies, including the large and well-known Lyon study. In that study, it was found that in individuals who had already suffered a first heart attack, the Mediterranean diet produced a 70 percent decrease in rates of a second heart attack over the subsequent four years.

Only a few studies have looked specifically at the effect of the Mediterranean diet on the risk of developing dementia. However, the data strongly suggest that the diet reduces that risk. In a study performed at the Columbia University Medical Center, the Mediterranean diet was found to reduce the risk of developing Alzheimer's dementia by up to 40 percent. Similar results were found in an Italian study of the effects of the Mediterranean diet on Alzheimer's and vascular dementias.

It is fortunate that the Mediterranean style of eating is not only healthy but is also among the most delicious cuisines in the world. There are hundreds of cookbooks and meal-planning books built around the Mediterranean style of eating. They are in every library and bookstore.

REACH AND MAINTAIN YOUR IDEAL BODY WEIGHT

To a large degree, obesity is seen as a risk factor for dementia because it is so closely associated with metabolic syndrome, heart disease, and diabetes. However, there are studies showing that obesity itself may increase the risk of dementia independently from the other factors. Thus, an important part of reducing the risk of dementia is to reach and maintain your ideal body weight.

Your ideal weight depends primarily upon your sex and height. If you are a man your ideal weight can be calculated by assuming 106 pounds for your first five feet of height plus 6 pounds for each additional inch. If you are a woman, assume 100 pounds for your first five feet of height, and add 5 pounds for each additional inch of height. If you are over fifty years of age, add an extra 10 pounds to obtain your ideal weight. There is also an adjustment for the size of your skeletal frame. If it is large, you add 10 pounds. If it is small, you subtract 10 pounds.

Regardless of what you eat, whether it is high fat, high protein, or high carbohydrate, the *only* way to lose weight is to consume fewer calories than your body uses. You must either decrease the amount of calories you consume, increase the number of calories you burn through exercise, or do both at the same time. Most people find that the latter method is the most successful.

Any diet that restricts calories will lead to weight loss. I have recommended the Mediterranean diet as the healthiest diet for most people to eat on a daily basis. However, the diet you choose to maintain your health need not be the same diet you use to lose excess pounds. Although weight loss is ultimately the result of using more calories than you burn, the types of food you eat can make losing weight easier.

Meals that are high in protein are more satisfying than meals high in carbohydrate. People eat less when their meal is rich in protein. Moreover, after a meal of protein, the next meal a person eats tends to be smaller than if their first meal had been high in carbohydrate. Because many of the amino acids in protein can be converted to glucose in the liver, a meal of protein stimulates release of insulin much like a meal of carbohydrate. However, protein acts like a very low-glycemic-index carbohydrate. It produces a long and sustained supply of blood glucose, which in turn causes a low, but long and sustained release of insulin. The insulin contributes to a feeling of satiety. Certain amino acids in protein, leucine in particular, may themselves generate a satiety effect.

Other hormones that affect hunger are affected differently by fat, carbohydrate, and protein. The gut hormone ghrelin increases appetite. Both protein and carbohydrate decrease blood levels of ghrelin, and in this way decrease feelings of hunger. However, whereas ghrelin levels quickly rebound after a meal rich in carbohydrate, they tend to stay low for hours after a meal of protein. This is one more reason that high protein meals tend to be more satisfying. Fat does not affect either insulin or ghrelin, but it does stimulate release of the appetite-suppressing hormone cholecystokinin. For these reasons, diets high in protein and healthy fat with low amounts of carbohydrate tend to be more effective and easier to stay on, at least for the first few months.

Foods that have a high glycemic index, that is, foods that quickly flood the bloodstream with sugar, can be satisfying for a brief period of time. Insulin, which is released into the blood after meals, not only lowers blood glucose, but also produces a satiety effect. That is, it stimulates areas of the brain to feel satisfied rather than hungry. However, after a meal of rapidly digested and absorbed carbohydrate, a large burst of insulin is secreted, which quickly lowers blood glucose back to normal. With glucose levels back to normal, insulin levels decrease and no longer provide any satiety effect.

In some cases, large amounts of insulin released in response to a sudden load of high-glycemic-index carbohydrate can overshoot its goal of normalizing glucose, and within a few hours produce a lower than normal glucose level, or hypoglycemia. Hypoglycemia leads to food craving, which leads to binging and a vicious cycle of eating and hunger. Meals with complex carbohydrate, that is, low-glycemic-index carbohydrates that are slowly digested and only gradually increase blood glucose, do not cause a burst of insulin that can cause hypoglycemia. Complex carbohydrates cause a sustained level of glucose and a similarly sustained release of insulin that generates a longer lasting satiety signal in the brain. For successful dieting, it is best to increase intake of protein and healthy fat and to decrease intake of carbohydrate. The carbohydrates that are consumed should have a low glycemic index.

The most well-known high protein, high fat, and low carbohydrate diet is the Atkins diet. Initially, doctors were aghast at a diet that encouraged patients to eat as much bacon, eggs, steak, and other foods high in fat and protein as they wished. However, over the past ten years or so, a large number of studies have found that the Atkins diet is not only effective, but far less a danger than doctors had suspected. This is likely due to the fact that carbohydrate is the driving force behind many, if not most, instances of high cholesterol, high triglycerides, and high blood glucose, which in large part is simply metabolic syndrome. Many people find that they can lose weight more quickly and easily on the Atkins diet than other diets they have tried, and for this reason people should be encouraged to try the diet if they wish to do so. However, it must also be stated that the advantages of the Atkins diet tend to diminish with time. Although many people initially relish their freedom to eat as much steak, butter, and bacon as they wish, it isn't too many weeks before they are beside themselves craving a simple piece of French bread with their dinner. Thus, the ease with which they stay on their diet can soon be lost. Finally, while many studies show an enhanced ability to lose weight early in the Atkins diet, this advantage tends to disappear after a few months.

It is important to unburden yourself of the false notion that you can eat endless amounts of food on the Atkins style of diet and still lose weight. That you might eat as much as you want and still lose weight can be true only in that you will likely want to eat less because your appetite is reduced by the high protein and high fat diet. There may be some unique physiological effects of the diet that can burn a few extra calories a bit faster, such as the phenomenon of uncoupling and enhancement of what is called thermogenesis. However, the contributions made by these effects are trivial. The Atkins diet does not allow you to escape the fundamental laws of physiology and biochemistry. If you consume more calories than you burn, you will gain, not lose weight.

If you do choose the Atkins style diet of high protein, high fat, low carbohydrate, keep in mind that good fats, such as olive oil and trans-fat-free margarine, can be used instead of butter, lard, and other fats high in saturated fat. There is no need to gorge yourself on beef steaks loaded with saturated fat, when salmon and other fish rich in healthy omega-3 fatty acids are so delicious. Instead of bacon or sausage with eggs for breakfast, kippers with your eggs may be just as enjoyable. Low-fat cheese can reduce the saturated fat burden, and choices of lean meats such as buffalo rather than beef can also improve the mix of fatty acids in your weight loss diet.

The body is extraordinarily efficient in using calories. The average adult needs only the number of calories in a large apple, about 150, to run a mile. If you changed nothing in your life except for adding the running of a mile every day for a month, you would burn an extra 4500 calories. With ten calories of energy in each gram of fat in your body, this would amount to burning 450 grams of fat, or about one pound of weight loss over that month of time. Yes, it is disappointing. However, as I have alluded to in several sections of this book, exercise involves more than simple burning of calories. Including exercise as part of a weight loss program makes it easier for people to stay with their reduced calorie diets. In many, though not all people, exercise appears to reduce hunger during dieting. Some of this effect of exercise is hormonal. For example, there is evidence that moderate degrees of both resistance and aerobic exercise decrease levels of the hormone ghrelin, which in turn would tend to decrease appetite. Regular exercise also tends to increase baseline levels of the hormone adiponectin, which would also result in decreases in appetite. Women who are athletic and active tend to have higher metabolic rates than women who do not exercise. A higher metabolic rate, which is the amount of energy an individual burns while simply at rest, is associated with less difficulty in reaching and maintaining ideal weight. Of course, weight loss is only one of many reasons to exercise.

EXERCISE YOUR BODY

Exercise reduces the likelihood of heart disease, diabetes, metabolic syndrome, and obesity, which all increase the likelihood of dementia. One would thus expect that exercise might reduce the risk of dementia. There is an abundance of evidence that this is the case. Exercise in young and mid adulthood has far-reaching effects in preventing dementia in later years. Adults who are regularly active in sports or light exercise, such as walking or gardening, are less likely to develop Alzheimer's dementia when they become elderly than are people who do not exercise. Adults sixty-five years of age and above who have normal cognitive function show less likelihood of developing Alzheimer's dementia if they exercise at least three times a week. In some cases, this was vigorous exercise, such as running or weight training; however, walking, swimming, hiking, and casual bicycling were equally effective.

In a study of still relatively young adults, fifty years of age and older, who were already diagnosed with MCI, it was found that walking briskly for fifty minutes three days a week significantly improved their cognitive function, and this improvement was maintained over the three years of the study. It is never too late to benefit from the ability of exercise to hold off dementia. People as old as their mid eighties who have retained normal cognitive function are more likely to continue to possess good function over the next few years if they exercise. In patients already diagnosed with Alzheimer's dementia, even those with moderate or even severe degrees of illness, decline in cognitive function is slowed down by as little as two hours of mild exercise a week. The exercise can be as simple as walking and stretching exercises.

Exercise might reduce the risk of dementia by means other than improving predisposing conditions such as metabolic syndrome and heart disease. For example, moderate intensity exercise programs lead to reduced resting levels of the stress hormone cortisol. Exercise is also known to increase levels of the growth factor BDNF in the brain and the blood. BDNF stimulates the dendrites of neurons to grow, and it is thought to be an important substance in learning, in the maintenance of existing neurons, and the growth of new neurons in the process of neurogenesis. BDNF and neurogenesis are also thought to be important in maintaining mood, which may be at least one reason that exercise is also useful in the treatment of major depression. Evidence from animal studies shows that young animals produce more BDNF in their brains in response to exercise than do old animals. Nonetheless, though age limits, it does not prevent the beneficial effects of exercise on BDNF from occurring in the brain.

Exercise also reduces inflammation and oxidative stress in the brain, which can increase deposition of amyloid. Studies in animals given human genes for amyloid precursor protein have shown that exercise slows down the accumulation of amyloid in brain tissue. Inflammation is also known to blunt the stimulating effects of growth factors in the brain; thus, exercise may both stimulate BDNF as well as free it from some inhibitory effects. Exercise increases blood flow to the brain during the activity itself. More significantly, it may also improve the blood supply to the brain such that benefits are also enjoyed between exercise sessions. The brain retains its normal volume and resists the usual shrinkage of aging in people who exercise regularly. This may be due to increases in blood supply, with more blood vessels and capillaries, but may also reflect better maintenance of gray matter.

Studies have shown that any kind of exercise can be beneficial to prevent dementia or, in people already suffering from the illness, to slow its progression. Nonetheless, there are some exercises that may be more helpful than others in their ability to improve and maintain cognitive function. Aerobic exercise, if it can be performed safely, may be the best form of exercise. Aerobic does not necessarily refer to how strenuous an exercise is. In fact, the phrase "aerobic exercise" was originally coined to distinguish it from exercise so vigorous that muscles deplete their supply of oxygen and are forced to "burn" fuel without oxygen, or anaerobically. Weight lifting or sprinting at top speed can produce such anaerobic conditions in muscle tissue. Simply stated, aerobic exercise is any activity that increases your body's demand on oxygen. It is generally taken to mean increases in oxygen demand that are long and strong enough to stimulate the heart, muscles, and metabolic systems of the body to make subtle changes in preparation for the next session of exercise. These changes add up to produce what is called conditioning. A simple rule of thumb that I tell my patients is that if your heart rate increases, you are breathing more heavily, and you begin to break a sweat, but you still have enough wind to be able to carry on a conversation with someone else, you are probably engaging in a helpful form of aerobic exercise.

Aside from the aerobic quality of exercise, another important component is the degree to which using your mind is incorporated into the exercise. Thus dancing, which requires awareness of orientation in space, balance, remembering steps, and paying attention to rhythm, is more beneficial than simply walking briskly. Similarly, playing the piano is more beneficial than exercises that might demand similar effort to simply move and stretch the upper extremities.

Of course, exercise puts demands on the heart, blood vessels, bones, and muscles that can cause harm if not performed in a safe and well-controlled manner. Thus, particularly for individuals who are elderly, ill, or simply poorly conditioned due to inactivity, it is essential to seek the advice of a doctor or a physical therapist prior to embarking on an exercise program.

GET A GOOD NIGHT'S SLEEP

Insufficient sleep and irregular sleep schedules both contribute to stress, metabolic syndrome, mood disturbances, and increased risk of dementia. Studies have shown that after a week of restricting sleep to only four hours a night, people begin to show evidence of decreases in sensitivity to insulin. Prolonged periods of such inadequate sleep increase the risk of obesity, metabolic syndrome, and diabetes type 2.

There is no absolute number of hours a person must sleep. A long-held notion has been that eight hours of sleep per night is ideal for adults. In fact, there is evidence that people who live longer and perform well tend to need only six hours of sleep per night. However, it is very unlikely that simply limiting yourself to six hours of sleep would benefit you if it is contrary to your nature.

The best measure of whether or not you are getting enough sleep is how you feel from day to day. If it is difficult to get up in the morning, if you tend to nod off during your day if you sit down in a comfortable chair, or if you simply feel tired throughout the day, it is likely that you are not getting enough sleep at night. Another indication of whether or not you are getting enough sleep is how long you tend to sleep on weekends when you have no obligation to get up. If weekday and weekend sleep times greatly differ, it is likely that you are not getting enough sleep. If you are awakened every morning by an alarm clock, you are probably not getting enough sleep.

Insufficient sleep can be due to many different causes. Many people have difficulty getting to sleep. Often this is due to poor sleep habits, or what is often referred to by the rather quaint name of "sleep hygiene." Doctors who specialize in sleep medicine have established some basic principles of sleep hygiene that can help a person get to sleep and form healthy sleep patterns. By and large, the advice that any sleep specialist will give you will consist of variations of the same following hints:

- Get up and go to bed at the same time every day.
- Refrain from exercise for at least four hours before bedtime.
- Stay away from caffeine and nicotine for at least four to six hours before bed. Alcohol may lull you to sleep, but as it wears off, your sleep will be disrupted. It should be avoided as well.
- Have a light snack before bed. Some warm milk, rich in the sleep-inducing amino acid tryptophan, is an age-old and still helpful pleasure.
- A cool room is more conducive to sleep than a hot room.
- Keep your bedroom dark and quiet for sleep. If it is impossible to keep the room quiet (e.g., if you have a snoring spouse!), consider earplugs. White noise machines can be helpful to mask environmental noises.
- If you can't fall asleep within twenty minutes, get up and do something relaxing until you feel sleepy.
- Use your bed for only sleeping and sex.

Modern society places great demands upon our time, and our sleep is often a casualty of irregular work hours and shifting work schedules. Studies have shown that work schedules other than the usual "nine to five" can be quite stressful. Surprisingly, working at night or shifting week to week from daytime to nighttime work schedules can increase rates of obesity, high levels of cholesterol, hyperglycemia, insulin resistance, and all of the other components of metabolic syndrome. When offered a good job, particularly when the job market is tough, most people set aside their concerns for how the job will affect their sleep schedule. Nonetheless, it is likely worthwhile to accept a job that pays slightly less if it is easier on your ability to get a full night's sleep on a regular basis.

Difficulty getting to sleep and staying asleep can also be signs of a psychiatric illness such as major depression or bipolar affective disorder. If difficulty sleeping is accompanied by sadness, mood swings, changes in appetite, loss of pleasure, hopelessness, or social withdrawal, it is possible that such an illness is contributing to the insomnia. A hallmark of sleep that is disturbed by major depression is early morning awakening. It is not uncommon for people to have difficulty getting to sleep, and then to awaken at three or four o'clock in the morning unable to return to sleep. When in the "up" phase, individuals with the various forms of bipolar affective disorder experience sleeplessness or not needing to sleep for days at a time. People who suffer bipolar affective disorder can be exquisitely sensitive to irregular sleep schedules. I and other psychiatrists have noted that many episodes of mild or even severe mania can be cut short simply by getting the patient to sleep well for several consecutive nights. I strongly advise people diagnosed with bipolar affective disorder to look for jobs with standard working hours and to avoid graveyard shifts or work hours that shift from week to week. If you suspect that symptoms of major depression or bipolar affective disorder may be a part of your inability to sleep, you should speak with your doctor about it.

GET YOUR SLEEP APNEA DIAGNOSED AND TREATED

Sleep apnea is a very common problem that is growing in frequency along with rates of obesity and metabolic syndrome. Sleep apnea is generally defined as cessation of breathing during sleep for periods of ten seconds or more. It deprives the brain of oxygen as well as sleep. Sleep apnea places great stress on the brain and body, and it is a major risk factor for Alzheimer's and vascular dementias.

Sleep apnea should be suspected anytime you suffer the symptoms of insufficient sleep. If you snore in your sleep and have risk factors for sleep apnea, which are obesity and metabolic syndrome, the likelihood of your suffering sleep apnea increases. It is essential that you see your doctor about this possibility. In some cases it may be possible to perform a simple screening test at home with a small device called a recording oximeter. This instrument clamps comfortably on your finger and measures and records your blood oxygen level and heart rate for the entire night. Alternatively, or subsequently to confirm suspicious findings by oximetry, your doctor may want a full battery of tests in a sleep lab. The advantage of a sleep lab study is that other conditions such as restless legs, central sleep apnea, or primary sleep disorders can be diagnosed. It is also possible in a sleep lab to immediately address the problem of obstructive sleep apnea by testing the effectiveness of pressurized breathing devices called CPAP or BIPAP. In some cases, sleep apnea can be treated by devices in the mouth that push the lower jaw forward and open up the airway in back of the tongue. It is not unusual that sleeping on your side rather your back and/or losing extra weight relieves the problems of sleep apnea.

There are not yet any medications approved to help reduce the severity of sleep apnea. However, there are some medications that seem to increase the ability of the brain to maintain tone in the muscles of the tongue. When these muscles relax, the tongue tends to fall back into the throat and block the airway. It is interesting that one of the types of medications that improves sleep apnea in laboratory studies is the cholinesterase inhibitor physostigmine. As you may recall, cholinesterase inhibitors are the medications that are approved by the FDA to treat dementia. Sleep apnea is extremely common among people who suffer Alzheimer's dementia, and there are experts who believe that a significant part of the therapeutic effect of cholinesterase inhibitors is some relief from sleep apnea.

AVOID ENVIRONMENTAL CONTRIBUTORS TO DEMENTIA

Along with being careful to eliminate unhealthy foods from our diet, such as those high in sugar and saturated fats, it is also important to avoid the many other toxic and injurious substances in the environment to reduce our risk of developing dementia. Many toxins are present in the food we eat, the water we drink, and the air we breathe. They are also present in the form of radioactivity from radon gas and electromagnetic radiation from the electronic and communication devices that are so much a part of the modern lifestyle.

As much as is possible and practical, eat fresh organic food. Avoid food and drink stored in plastic and cans, as these are the products that tend to contain BPA, that is, bisphenol A. Food free of pesticides and other agricultural chemicals is safer. In fact, when fruits and vegetables must fend for themselves, they increase their content of potentially beneficial substances like resveratrol, which they produce to protect themselves from molds, fungi, and other organisms. If you can't find or afford organically grown fruit and vegetables, at least make sure they are washed well with suitable cleanser before eating them.

Trans fats are sometimes considered an unhealthy food, but they are best described as contaminants. They are the result of the food industry tinkering with oil to artificially improve the creaminess, "mouth feel," and other characteristics of food. They cause a variety of problems that further the progress of metabolic syndrome. Consuming trans fatty acids increases the risk of heart attack. It has been estimated that every 5 gram increase in daily intake of trans fatty acid increases the risk of coronary artery disease by 25 percent. A meal of French fries and a deep-fried filet of chicken at a fast food restaurant may contain over 5.5 grams of trans fatty acid. Trans fats increase the risk of all forms of dementia by increasing the likelihood of metabolic syndrome and cardiovascular disease. Stay away from this poison.

If you live in an area that is heavily industrialized, you may want to have your water checked for common contaminants. Among the contaminants most frequently found in groundwater close to hazardous waste sites are the elements arsenic, cadmium, and lead. There are also a number of toxic industrial solvents, including benzene, toluene, and trichloroethylene, that have found their way into our drinking water. All of these substances, particularly lead and the solvent trichloroethylene, have been associated with cognitive dysfunction and dementia. There is no compelling reason to fear fluoride from drinking water or aluminum from soda cans. However, there may be reasonable concern about frequent drinking out of plastic bottles that contain the substance BPA, which has been found to cause brain damage in monkeys. It is not known if we consume amounts of BPA sufficient enough to cause damage. However, many such substances accumulate in the fat, and over time the body's burden may be substantial. It remains to be determined if cousins to BPA that are used in plastics, including phthalates, brominated diphenyl ethers, and perfluorinated organics (PFOCs), cause similar problems. As strongly as some have argued about mercury in dental fillings, the scientific data just isn't strong enough to suggest that you go to the extent of having those fillings replaced with plastic. Besides, at this point there is no certainty that the plastics used to replace the mercury amalgam are any safer. The best advice is to take care of your teeth. Avoiding tooth decay and gum disease will reduce your risk of dementia as well as needing fillings of any kind.

Studies show that air pollution in smoggy cities like Mexico City, and likely large American cites such as Los Angeles, can contribute to dementia. If practical, you might consider moving to a smaller city or town with cleaner air. Of course, air pollution is not always obvious, nor is it found solely in heavily industrialized areas. Radon gas, which is known to cause lung cancer and suspected of increasing the risk of dementia, can be found in high concentration throughout many rural areas in the United States. You may need to check with the county health department to learn the levels of these contaminants in your present location or in areas you are considering. If you are at high risk for exposure to these substances, consider air purifiers in your home. If radon is a problem, install exhaust fans to limit the amount of the radioactive gas that can build up in your basement or other low areas in your home.

The jury is still out concerning what if any risks are incurred by placing a cell phone next to your head for what may be hours a day. However, there are many easy ways that this danger can be reduced without doing away with this device that has become a modern necessity. The potential danger a cell phone poses from the extremely low frequency electromagnetic field (ELF-EMF) it generates is dramatically reduced by simply moving it farther away from your ear. They can be placed in speaker phone mode or earphones can be plugged into them to keep the phone and its antenna in your hand and away from your head. Blow dryers with their heat coils and rapidly spinning electric motors are also strong sources of ELF-EMF radiation. If you must use one, keep it as far away from your head as you can. The danger is greatly diminished with distance.

SUPPLEMENTATION WITH VITAMINS, HERBS, AND NUTRACEUTICALS

In the chapter on supplementation with vitamins, herbs, and nutraceuticals, I discussed a long list of substances that can be taken in addition to a healthy diet and other components of a healthy lifestyle to reduce your risk of developing dementia. What is most important to convey to you is that there is no reason to start taking *all* of the substances I discussed under the false impression that if one is good, ten must be better. Many have similar or at least overlapping effects, and to take a large number of these supplements in willy-nilly fashion would be redundant and very expensive. Combinations of these supplements should be chosen systematically to benefit from a specific set of effects and to suit individual needs, tastes, preferences, and pocketbooks.

Before going into specifics, I should begin by advising everyone to start with a single, once-a-day multiple vitamin and mineral supplement. Doctors and nutritionists agree that, ideally, all vitamins and minerals should be supplied by a healthy diet. However, in real life this cannot be depended upon. There is absolutely no danger in taking such a supplement, and it will insure that you receive the minimal daily requirement of the critical vitamins and minerals.

The specific effects that one would hope to gain from a combination of supplements to decrease the risk of dementia include antioxidant effects, anti-inflammatory effects, stimulation of neuron growth factors such as

BDNF, decreases in production and accumulation of sticky, beta amyloid protein, enhancement of acetylcholine activity, and decrease in the manifestations of metabolic syndrome, which would include stabilization of blood sugar levels, improvement in serum cholesterol and other lipids, normalization of blood pressure, and decreases in insulin resistance. There are also some supplements with unique effects that are of benefit in special circumstances.

The most prudent approach to supplementation is to take only what you need to add up to good coverage in all of the areas I've noted above. For example, one of many good combinations would be alpha-lipoic acid, ashwagandha, and huperzine. Another would be curcumin, grape seed extract, and sage.

In most cases, a single multiple-vitamin-and-mineral pill will not provide you with an optimal quantity of vitamins C, D, or E. Thus, I would advise everyone to add to the multiple-vitamin-and-mineral pills, 400 milligrams (mg) of vitamin C, 400 to 800 IUs of vitamin D, and 200 to 400 units of vitamin E in the form of natural, mixed tocopherols, on a daily basis. The omega 3 fatty acids EPA and DHA in fish oil are so beneficial and so likely to be deficient in the modern diet, that I advise everyone to take 2 to 3 grams of fish oil a day.

Vitamin B_{12} is critical for maintaining normal brain function. If you eat meat, eggs, or dairy, and normal blood levels confirm that you have no trouble absorbing the vitamin, then it is not necessary to supplement your diet with B_{12} tablets or shots. If you have been found to have low vitamin B_{12} levels, then 1mg (1000 micrograms) of it by mouth is sufficient to give a normal blood level of the vitamin, even if you have no production of intrinsic factor in the stomach.

One mg of folic acid provides a good supply of this critical vitamin, particularly if tests have shown you to have low or marginal levels. I have often suggested to my elderly patients with marginal folate levels to use a prenatal vitamin tablet as their daily multi-vitamin supplement. Prenatal vitamins are rich in folic acid, as it helps reduce the risk of certain birth defects.[1]

There are many substances that are produced in the body that predictably fall in concentration as we age. Everyone would benefit from their supplementation. Melatonin has many excellent properties that can help prevent dementia, which has led me to recommend using it as a preventa-

---

1. Some of my patients' inquiries about prenatal vitamins have stimulated a number of interesting comments from puzzled drugstore pharmacists. I say, "Keep them guessing."

tive measure. Around the age of sixty, people begin to show decreases in the amount of melatonin they produce and release during the night hours. Thus, I strongly suggest that anyone approaching the age of sixty take 3 to 5 mg of a reputable brand of melatonin every evening. DHEA is another natural substance in the body whose concentrations begin to drop as we age. As can be seen in the table in chapter 6, DHEA offers many benefits that could be of use for the prevention of dementia. Women who take DHEA often have a significant increase in blood levels of testosterone, which is associated with increased sex drive. Both men and women may experience improvement in mood with DHEA supplementation. Thus, despite some admittedly disappointing experimental data on the ability of DHEA to prevent dementia, I don't discourage adding 50 mg of DHEA a day.

I have also discussed several supplements that are best used by individuals with special situations and needs. Carnosine is a molecule that helps prevent the chemical bonding of sugar to protein that results in advanced glycation endproducts, or AGEs. AGEs are directly responsible for some damage in the body, such as cataracts in the eyes that rob elderly people of their sight. They also stimulate inflammatory responses in brain tissue that contribute to the neurodegenerative process of dementia. People who eat meat are usually able to get enough carnosine in their diet. A very similar substance called anserine is supplied in diets that include ocean fish. However, I strongly recommend that vegetarians supplement their diet with a gram of carnosine each day.

Chromium is found in egg yolk, meats, cereal grains, brewer's yeast, and spices. The consensus among nutritionists is that most people obtain sufficient chromium from their diet. However, because chromium is so very important in maintaining the body's sensitivity to insulin, I recommend 200 to 400 micrograms of supplemental chromium picolinate a day for anyone with signs of metabolic syndrome. Those signs include high blood pressure, high fasting blood glucose, high triglycerides, low good HDL cholesterol, and abdominal obesity. These signs will need to be confirmed by your doctor or other health care provider. Anyone who has already been diagnosed with diabetes type 2 should also take chromium, as the resistance to insulin persists even after the pancreas has stopped being able to produce sufficient levels of the hormone. Alpha-lipoic acid, which is helpful in anyone, is also a substance natural to the body and particularly useful in individuals with metabolic syndrome. It is also helpful for the neuropathic pain that afflicts sufferers of diabetes.

Co-enzyme Q10 is a natural substance in the body, and there is usually little reason to suspect that there are insufficient quantities in the body. However, the "statin" family of medicines that is prescribed to slow down the body's production of cholesterol also reduce the amount of CoQ10 that is produced. Anyone taking a statin should also be taking supplemental CoQ10. There are also known to be certain neurological diseases that arise from deficient mitochondrial activity that respond to treatment with supplemental CoQ10. Many of these, such as MELAS syndrome, chronic progressive external opthalmoplegia, and others are quite rare. However, some of these illnesses present with dementia as a component, and these may show some improvement with CoQ10 treatment. There has been some suspicion that Parkinson's disease and Lewy body dementia may arise from mitochondrial dysfunction in some people. However, there is little evidence that statin drugs make Parkinson's disease worse or that the illness improves after addition of CoQ10.

Red yeast rice is a natural form of statin that reduces the production of CoQ10 in a manner similar to what is seen with prescribed statins. If you are not taking a statin, you may want to consider red yeast rice. However, first discuss it with your doctor, and if you do start it, add supplementary CoQ10.

Idebenone is essentially a man-made form of CoQ10. It acts as a powerful antioxidant, which alone might be sufficient reason to add it as a supplement. What is most remarkable about idebenone is that under conditions of low oxygen, such as might be found in sleep apnea, heart failure, or chronic lung conditions such as emphysema, it is more efficient than CoQ10 in producing energy in the mitochondria. In fact, several studies suggest that while idebenone remains active in hypoxic states, the activity of CoQ10 "short circuits" and acts to trigger inflammatory processes. Thus, this leads me to recommend idebenone supplementation to anyone with sleep apnea, emphysema, COPD, congestive heart failure, or other illnesses that cause chronically low blood oxygen.

It is now well recognized by scientists that inflammation plays an important role in the process of neurodegeneration in dementia. This fact came to light largely because of the discovery that people who took ibuprofen and related medications on a daily basis to treat pain had a reduced risk of developing Alzheimer's dementia. Ibuprofen is an excellent anti-inflammatory. However, it turns out that ibuprofen may help reduce the risk of dementia by several different mechanisms. Anyone who wants to avoid dementia who also has evidence of an inflammatory state, such as an elevated C-reactive protein level, should certainly be taking ibuprofen daily. In fact, I would go so far as to say that unless you have a good reason to avoid ibuprofen, you should go ahead and take it anyway. The problem with ibuprofen is that it can irritate the stomach, contribute to ulcers, and exacerbate bleeding disorders. Thus, as I have emphasized throughout this section, speak to your doctor before starting on ibuprofen.

Vinpocetine is known to relax the walls of small arteries and allow more blood flow. It has been found to improve cognitive function in people who have suffered strokes or have been shown to have some sort of vascular insufficiency. It does not appear to offer great benefits for Alzheimer's or other forms of neurodegenerative dementia. However, it may be of benefit in people diagnosed with vascular dementia. Before you start idebenone or vinpocetine, be certain to discuss it with your doctor.

Garlic is very good for you, as are sage, rosemary, turmeric (which is the source of curcumin), black pepper (rich in chromium), and a number of other spices. However, remember that these can be added in more economical and tasteful fashion by using them liberally when you cook. These aromatic and tasty spices get some of their characteristics from polyphenols that often have antioxidant and other useful characteristics. You might also enjoy your morning coffee or green tea knowing that it is helping to protect your brain. Drink it with a piece of sugarless dark chocolate.

REDUCE STRESS

Stress increases blood levels of the hormone cortisol. High levels of cortisol antagonize the effects of insulin and accelerate deposition of visceral fat, both of which contribute to metabolic syndrome and diabetes. High levels of cortisol also contribute to major depression and obesity. All of those conditions are major risk factors for dementia.

There are many ways by which cortisol can initiate and accelerate neurodegenerative processes in the brain. In animal studies, administration of the rodent stress hormone corticosterone increases deposits of abnormal forms of amyloid and tau protein, just as is seen in the brains of patients with Alzheimer's dementia. In primates, cortisol inhibits the process of neurogenesis and thus prevents replacement of neurons in the adult brain. It also inhibits dendritic branching, which supports learning, memory, and processing of complex thoughts. Thus, it is not surprising that studies have found elderly people with the highest cortisol levels are also the ones most likely to develop dementia. A recent study published in the journal *Neurology* discovered that people over the age of seventy-five who were free of dementia at the beginning of the study were 50 percent less likely to develop dementia over the subsequent six years if they described themselves as relaxed, calm, and self-satisfied.

There are many techniques to relieve stress and reduce levels of cortisol. For example, reductions in serum or salivary cortisol have been reported during listening to music. Classical music has been found to improve cognitive performance not only in healthy, elderly subjects, but also in patients with Alzheimer's dementia. In fact, in one study, patients with moderate to severe dementia who were exposed daily to classical music were better able to maintain their cognitive function over a two-year period than were similar patients who did not receive music as therapy.

It isn't known if music offers adults in midlife any protection from developing dementia. Certainly, the calming effects of music offer stress reduction and improvement in mood that are known to reduce the risk of developing dementia over time. It is interesting, or at least amusing, that scientists have discovered that even young adult mice show improvement in cognitive function after listening to slow, soothing music six hours a day over three weeks. Those mice learned tasks more quickly, and hippocampal levels of the important neural growth factor BDNF were increased. I keenly suspect, and there is some experimental evidence to support, that listening to *any* type of music, whether classical, country, or even rock 'n' roll, can have a calming effect if it is the type of music the individual enjoys.

Meditation also reduces serum levels of cortisol. Meditation calms the mind, reduces stress, and improves mood. A sophisticated study recently performed at Emory University showed that habitual practice of Zen meditation not only improved attention in elderly subjects, but also helped maintain the volume of gray matter in an area of the brain called the putamen.[2] The putamen is an area known to be involved in consciously paying attention to the environment, and it is known to shrink in size as people age.

Yoga, tai chi, progressive relaxation, laughter, spending time in nature, and having a companion dog or cat reduce cortisol. People with spiritual convictions, derived from organized religions or not, have lower levels of cortisol than those who do not. Many of these additions to daily life have also been found to reduce the risk of dementia or to improve the function of people already diagnosed with the condition. It hasn't been proven that reductions in levels of cortisol are responsible for the beneficial effects of the practices noted above. The scientific studies that come closest to showing that specifically reducing cortisol activity can improve cognitive function in dementia are preliminary studies evaluating the effects of mifepristone, a

---

2. To the best of my knowledge, no one has yet trained mice to sit in lotus position and meditate to see if that improves their memory. However, I am eagerly awaiting results of such a study.

drug that blocks the effects of cortisol. Patients with Alzheimer's dementia who receive mifepristone over time have been found to preserve cognitive function longer than those who do not.

All in all, it is clear that high cortisol levels contribute to the development of Alzheimer's dementia, whereas many relaxing, enjoyable activities offer benefits to cognitive performance. Thus, stress reduction should be included in any program intended to reduce the risk of developing dementia.

TREAT DEPRESSION AND OTHER PSYCHIATRIC DISORDERS

Major depression and other mood disorders, as well as anxiety disorders, are important risk factors in developing dementia. People with a long history of depression have roughly twice the risk of developing Alzheimer's dementia as those who do not. Dementia appears at an earlier age in people with depression, and it leads them to earlier placement in nursing homes.

Depression is not just thoughts. It is a biological phenomenon. The abnormal physiology of depression reaches deeply into the brain, and its effects can be observed in increases in amyloid plaques and neurofibrillary tangles. Depression also increases the risks of metabolic syndrome, cardiovascular disease, and diabetes, which, in turn, each greatly increase the risk of developing dementia. Stress can increase the risk of depression, but depression also increases the amount of stress and blood level of cortisol that people are exposed to over their lifetimes. People with chronic depression develop poor eating habits and exercise less often. Depression is associated with poor sleep, obesity, and sleep apnea. A lifelong battle with depression also means lack of motivation and lost opportunities to pursue what life has to offer. It may mean less challenging jobs or a failure to pursue a higher level of education. It results in social isolation and failure to progress through the stages of life that are necessary to build a foundation of security and contentment in old age.

Although major depression is an important risk factor for metabolic syndrome and cardiovascular disease, it is important to point out that other mood disorders, such as bipolar affective disorder, and anxiety disorders, such as social phobia, PTSD, and generalized anxiety, can also increase the risk of those conditions. They must be recognized and successfully treated to reduce the risk of dementia.

As a psychiatrist, I daily see patients who suffer mild to severe degrees of depression. Many people resist the suggestion of taking pills, and it is important to note that successful treatment of depression and other mood disorders does not have to include medication. One thing that I have come to realize over my years of practicing psychiatry is that simply being able to tell one's story to someone else can be the remedy for many cases of depression. It doesn't matter if a person is a shoe salesman or the CEO of a major financial institution. We all need to tell our story. It is tragic that our modern society leaves little room or opportunity for this simple but profound act of human communication. It restores our dignity, and breaks through barriers of isolation, guilt, resentment, and doubt. I believe that 90 percent of our anguish and emotional pain is our feeling unable to tell someone else what is really on our minds. It must also be recognized that while the brain is one of the most important organs in the body, it is nonetheless part of the body and subject to its rules. A healthy diet, stress reduction, exercise, and restful sleep strengthens and heals the brain, and can play an important part in relieving needless anxieties and episodes of feeling low. Relying on medication when those simple and natural means might be effective is imprudent.

With the above statements having been made, I must state that in some cases, the burden of severe, long-standing depression takes its toll on the chemistry of the brain and body, and substantive measures must be taken to return the body to a healthy state. Some people are biologically predisposed to mood disorders, and the most direct route to restoring their mental health and well-being is by helping re-equilibrate the brain with medications.

Many people are relieved to learn that starting an antidepressant does not necessarily mean that they will have to take that medicine for the rest of their lives. The rule of thumb is that after a person's first episode of serious depression that requires medication, it is entirely reasonable to taper and stop that medication after the person has been feeling well for six to eight months. If this person has stopped medication and later has a second episode of severe depression requiring medication, it is still possible to go off that medication after ten to twelve months of feeling well. It is generally thought that a third episode of severe depression requiring medication means that a person has a virtual 100 percent chance of having yet another episode of depression if he or she stops the antidepressant, and he or she is best advised to continue it. There are few medications of any kind more dangerous than staying severely depressed. In any case, modern antidepressants are quite safe, and there is little reason to fear taking such a medication for years or, if need be, for the rest of your life.

It is important to state that there is no compelling evidence that long-term use of antidepressants can cause dementia. There may even be some hitherto unexpected extra benefits of antidepressants. Several studies now show that certain antidepressants, including fluoxetine (Prozac), paroxetine (Paxil), citalopram (Celexa, Lexapro), and imipramine reduce the accumulation of amyloid and hyperphosphorylated tau protein in the brain tissue of experimental animals genetically predisposed to a brain disorder similar to Alzheimer's dementia. Those effects of the medications appear to be due to direct effects on the metabolism of the APP, or amyloid precursor protein, and not to relief of depression.

If you feel depressed or anxious for much of the day for an extended period of time, mention this to your doctor. There is no need to feel embarrassed or ashamed. Chances are good that doctors themselves have been treated or counseled in some fashion for their own experiences of depression, and they will know exactly what you are talking about.

EXERCISE YOUR MIND

When we are young, from kindergarten through college, our brains are stimulated by learning new skills, being exposed to new things, and being surrounded by interesting people with which to interact. As adults, we keep our minds sharp through the intellectual demands of our occupations and professions. Studies show that interesting, challenging jobs during adulthood reduce the risk of developing dementia. Certainly, some jobs are more stimulating than others. Taking orders that sound the same all day from behind a fast food counter, jobs on assembly lines, and other types of repetitive work are the mind-numbing work-life equivalent of a steady diet of white bread and cotton candy. However, a person doesn't have to be a lawyer or a rocket scientist to have mentally challenging work to do. Carpenters, plumbers, teachers, police officers, and mechanics all use their minds constantly to solve unique mathematical, spatial, logical, and social problems that arise throughout their workday. If you are young enough to still be working, it is important to seek work that is challenging. Keep learning and keep stimulating your mind. There is strong evidence that along with a good education in childhood and young adulthood, a challenging job during one's career helps build what is referred to as "cognitive reserve." It is not unlike the idea of a spare tire. Even when dementia does emerge, extra brain circuits built through years of mental stimulation seem to allow a person to limp around the brain damage.

There is growing evidence that studying, learning, and putting the brain to work help improve and maintain cognitive function regardless of a person's age. Animal studies have shown that when placed into a new environment with new things to learn and experience, even "elderly" mice have increases in the number of neurons in the hippocampus due to stimulation of neurogenesis. Using the brain turns on the basic housekeeping and maintenance functions in nerve cells and stimulates growth of the dendritic processes that neurons send out to contact other neurons. The information that is learned can be used to later solve similar problems.

I would encourage all people to keep working at their jobs as many years as they like if they enjoy it. Unfortunately, in our culture we are encouraged to retire from work in our mid sixties. If we do retire, we are thereafter faced with the problem of how to continue to engage our minds with stimulating, challenging experiences. Retirement is an excellent time to start adult education classes. Several studies have found that taking courses in midlife helps maintain verbal ability and memory as a person enters late life. Schaie determined that even individuals in their seventies and eighties can benefit from training in how best to solve problems, and these benefits can be observed years later.

Still, whether we are old or young, the best mental exercises are not performed in classrooms, but rather they are the ones that arise naturally out of doing interesting things with interesting people in the real world. Retirement allows some the opportunity to become politically active or to volunteer time in community efforts. Retirement can also provide the time to travel to interesting places and experience new things. We tend to underestimate how much of our minds are used in planning and preparing for travel. Travel itself, with the demands of schedules, reading maps and travel brochures, and learning what is necessary to know to get by in an unfamiliar environment and culture, is an excellent workout for the mind.

Socializing provides wonderful opportunities to stimulate the mind. Playing bridge or gin rummy with congenial friends once a week is wonderful mental exercise, especially if it is accompanied by lively conversation. The old men in the park playing dominoes with old friends are doing more than simply passing time. They are staying young. One of the most consistent findings in research is that people who maintain close friendships through adulthood and old age are most likely to avoid dementia. This is due to improvement in sense of well-being, relief from stress that isolation can bring, and the stimulation that one enjoys in interaction with other people.

Reading books and newspapers is wonderful mental exercise, as well as a way to stay current with world events. I strongly encourage it. By its very nature, reading books tends to isolate people if that's how they spend all their time. On the other hand, one of the best ways to exercise the brain and maintain the full range of cognitive function is to be a member of a book discussion club. This provides an avenue to read and enjoy books, as well as to socialize and discuss ideas with like-minded people.

Not surprisingly, sitting passively for hours in front of a television set not only lacks protective effects, but may actually be a risk factor for developing dementia. Although parents of teenagers have long suspected this to be the case, the adverse effects of television watching on cognitive function were discussed in a paper published in the prestigious *Proceedings of the National Academy of Sciences*. I must add, however, that a little television is harmless. Television can provide relaxation, news and current events, and, if thought-provoking programs are selected, it can be a source of some intellectual stimulation.

It is important not to neglect spatial, musical, and movement skills that are generally thought to be processed by the right hemisphere of the brain. Solving a jigsaw puzzle is a good exercise of visuospatial skills. Many interesting and pleasant conversations are held around the card table when a couple of friends are tackling a particularly difficult puzzle. Schaie notes that there is no better mental exercise than square dancing. Square dancing involves not only movement, orientation in space, and rhythm, but also remembering dance steps and melodies. Schaie notes that women, who are particularly prone to losing visuospatial skills after menopause, show significant improvement in laboratory tests of visuospatial function after several months of participating in square dancing or solving jigsaw puzzles. Of course, there is no better social involvement than dancing, whether, square, folk, or ballroom.

Just as supplementation with vitamins and minerals can be helpful to ensure that we receive an adequate supply of nutrients, I think it is quite reasonable to supplement our mental lives with tolerable doses of specific mental exercises, just to ensure that all aspects of our minds are being used, stimulated, and kept in good condition. There are many ways to supplement mental activity. Newspapers often have crossword puzzles, sudoku, or other types of brain teasers as a daily feature. Solving one of these puzzles can be an excellent way to ensure you are using your brain in a challenging fashion every day. There are also books full of puzzles and brain teasers that can challenge the mind. The best books of this sort present a variety of games and puzzles that can challenge and stimulate different aspects of mental activity, such as memory, using numbers, solving visual and spatial problems, or looking for hidden figures or words. Such books are available at local bookstores and through the Internet.

Of course, the Internet itself offers an astonishing array of games and brain teasers that can be used to supplement your mental exercise program.

The computer screen is particularly well suited to challenging memory with images to be remembered and later retrieved in what cognitive scientists call "matching to sample" tasks. Computers provide an endless variety of opportunities to play board and card games, either against the computer or real, living opponents on the Internet. Even the great workplace bugaboo, computer solitaire, can be used to stimulate thinking.

One of the best ways to challenge your mind and stimulate growth and maintenance of neurons and their dendrites is by doing new and different things with your mind. It can be as simple as doing some of your usual daily activities in different ways. For example, if you are right-handed, try feeding yourself or writing your shopping list with your left hand. Eat a meal with your eyes closed. After first taking care to remove sharp objects, rummage through a tool tray or kitchen "junk drawer" and identify objects by touch only. Spell words backward and perform arithmetic problems in your mind. Use your mind to visualize the streets and highways you use to drive to work or to your favorite restaurant. Visualize a tool, building, or kitchen utensil, and turn it in your mind's eye, imagining what it would look like from different angles. If you use your imagination, the list of such exercises you can contrive is endless. Just remember that exercises and games are merely fun and convenient supplements to brain activity. They are poor substitutes for interaction with people in interesting ways in the real world.

STAY SOCIALLY ACTIVE

The male orangutan is a solitary animal. He stays by himself, deep in the forest. He rarely interacts with other orangutans, except to bellow a warning to stay away. He seeks the company of the female orangutan only to mate. After mating, he quickly retreats back to his lair. A few women have described their husbands to me in this fashion. However, by and large, we humans are social animals. Unlike the male orangutan, who chooses isolation, for humans, isolation is the worst of punishments. When there is no other way left to control a hardened prisoner, the threat of solitary confinement may yet be an effective means to improve behavior.

Being alone is not necessarily a bad or troubling experience. We all need our "space." However, being lonely is both emotionally and physically distressing. Loneliness is associated not only with major depression, but also with high blood pressure, heart disease, high levels of cortisol, obesity, insulin resistance, poor sleep, and other dangerous physical manifestations.

We need other people to stimulate our minds and motivate us to act in the world. Without other people, we begin to withdraw and deteriorate.

Teaching and sharing the information we have gathered through our years is likely to be the very reason that we live as long as we do. Conversely, it stands to reason that sharing ourselves and our experiences in social situations is something that keeps us young and maintains our cognitive functions. This supposition is supported by a large medical literature. One of the most consistent findings in research into prevention of dementia is that maintaining social contacts with other people reduces the risk of developing dementia. Close friendships are particularly important. There is even data to suggest that having close confidants, people that we can freely speak our minds to, is as important as or even more important than maintaining family relationships. In this context, it is worth noting that most studies have not found marital status, that is, whether a person is married, divorced, or separated, to be a major factor in determining the risk for developing dementia. This rather surprising finding may be due to the fact that marriage can either be a blessing or a curse, depending on the quality of the relationship. Nonetheless, it has been found that those who never marry are at relatively high risk for dementia, as are people who have lost a spouse late in life. I think it is safe to conclude that a good marriage, where the spouse is also a friend and confidant, is the best of all possibilities.

One of the largest and most comprehensive studies of the effects of social activity on risk of dementia is the Honolulu-Asia Aging Study. In that study, just over 2,500 men were evaluated at ages between forty-five and sixty, and again twenty-three years later to determine what degree of social interaction they engaged in. These social interactions included marital status, living with extended family, having close friends, and being involved in community or political events. Such activity during midlife appeared to have minimal effect on the risk of later developing dementia. However, maintaining those social interactions in later life significantly improved the likelihood of remaining free of dementia. Another similar study found that elderly people who had little social contact with spouses, children, or neighbors suffered loss of memory at a rate twice that of those who maintained such social interaction. An interesting finding has been that people with large social networks can overcome some of the adverse effects of amyloid and neurofibrillary tangles in the brain. As has been found in people with good educations, it appears that people who are socially active can have better cognitive function than isolated individuals, despite having the same amount of neurodegenerative damage in their brain tissue.

GENERATIVITY, INTEGRITY, AND SPIRITUAL WELL-BEING

Sigmund Freud led science to the recognition that the human mind has great complexity and depth. Many factors mold and shape the mind, and many of our actions, decisions, and motivations take place subconsciously, below our awareness. We are indebted to Freud for his profound observations. However, many of his theories have become dated. For example, since Freud pondered the question "What do women want?", many scholarly, thoughtful, and articulate women have provided answers that did not occur to him. Often the answer has been, "We want what you want, Sigmund." Also, as Freud himself anticipated, an astounding amount of information has been learned about how the mind is rooted in neurochemical activity of the brain, and much of what Freud considered to be based in personality may in fact be secondary to genetic and environmental effects on brain chemistry. A major complaint about Freud's conceptualization of personality development has been his assumption that all of the important events that shape the mind and personality occur in childhood.

Erik Erikson was a student of art until he met Sigmund Freud's daughter, Anna, and became interested in psychoanalysis. He himself underwent psychoanalysis and went on to study at the Vienna Psychoanalytic Institute. One of Erikson's greatest accomplishments was to reconsider Freud's notions of the stages of human personality development and to conceive and build an expanded, more comprehensive view of human development that continues through adulthood and old age.

Erikson believed that the major task of middle age is to accomplish what he referred to as generativity. Generativity is the unselfish passing on of one's wisdom and resources to the younger generation and all future generations. For many people, this is the task of raising children, suffering their "leaving the nest," and then tending to grandchildren. For all people, particularly those who do not have children, generativity can be achieved by giving of themselves to students or young people in the community. It can also be achieved by working for the good of mankind, through invention, research, the arts, and social activism.

It is an unselfish relationship with the young that is the key to generativity. A successful relationship with a spouse is one founded on equality and reciprocity. However, the nurturance of children and other young people requires the capacity for true, unconditional love. Giving unconditional love and learning to accept the hurt and disappointment that can be felt when this love is denied or abused brings mellowing and humility. It lays a foundation for a sense of self-worth and accomplishment in being able to give back to the world and make it a better place for those to come.

The task of achieving generativity is often difficult, and it may culminate in what is often referred to as a "midlife crisis." Failure to achieve generativity leaves one in a state of what Erikson called stagnation. Stagnation may play out as a desperate striving to recapture an idealized youth. Instead of consolidating and reaping the harvest of long, loving relationships and the satisfaction of seeing one's children begin to flourish, the person unsuccessfully struggling with this stage of life may throw it all away for reckless exploits, sexual adventures, and shallow pursuits. However, this stage of life is an expected and difficult struggle, and some may need to experience, first-hand, such behavior before coming to grips with finding more substantial and age-appropriate means of "filling the empty space" and moving on. Besides which, expensive sports cars can be a lot of fun!

Generativity makes it possible, whereas stagnation makes it impossible, to progress to and through the final task of development. That final task is to find meaning and peace with one's self. Erikson referred to this as finding "integrity." This task generally presents itself at the difficult time in life when one is faced with letting go of much of what sustained one earlier in life. One's health and strength may be in decline. The power and responsibility that was worked for and enjoyed in the adult years has faded and been passed on to others. Siblings and friends are likely to have died, and it is time to fully come to terms with the fact that one's own life is limited. Successful performance of this task leads to a sense of fulfillment and satisfaction with what one has achieved in life. It includes the ability to forgive one's self for the mistakes made along the way and to fully appreciate the understanding that though we try our best, we are human and none of us reach perfection. It is the sense of spirituality that comes with seeing one's place in the world and in the great scheme of life. It is letting go and having faith that God or, as another might see it, the cycles of life and the universe, beyond our control or understanding, are doing their work as they should. Inability to find peace and contentment amidst the physical suffering and emotional losses of old age leads to despair. Despair leads to bitterness, dwelling in the past, suspicion, isolation, and depression. Despair exacerbates dementia.

Religious belief is by no means an antidote for dementia. However, organized religions, aside from all their faults, do provide structure for older adults to experience and be immersed in the teachings and comforts of faith. Ceremonies that provide direction and solemnity in the search for meaning and reunification with the eternal have evolved over many centuries. They should not be minimized or dismissed. Schaie himself has written on the subject of religious faith in old age, and was one of the editors of the book *Religious Influences on Health and Well-Being in the Elderly*. This book acknowledges and explores the fact that for the elderly, religious belief is a source of forgiveness, understanding, meaning in life, coping with loss, and, in more physiological terms, stress reduction. Scientific studies have been performed that showed that those with deeply held religious belief and dedication to spiritual practices, regardless of the kind, have a slower rate of cognitive decline when Alzheimer's dementia is diagnosed.

8

WHEN MEDICATION IS NECESSARY

If at all possible, it is best to prevent or treat dementia with healthy changes in lifestyle. But, realistically, this isn't always possible. In some cases, people are strongly predisposed to dementia or to the major risk factors for dementia. Many people already suffer some degree of dementia and need help. In such cases, medication can offer the easiest and most effective, albeit not risk free, means to reduce the risk of dementia or prevent it from rapidly getting worse.

In the United States there are only two basic types of medications that are approved by the FDA to treat dementia. One is the class of cholinesterase-inhibiting drugs, of which there are several different kinds, and the other is memantine (brand name Namenda). There are no drugs approved by the FDA to prevent the development of dementia, or to treat MCI, which is the mild loss of cognitive function that often precedes actual dementia.

PRESCRIPTION MEDICATIONS FOR DEMENTIA

The cholinesterase inhibitors were the first type of drug available to treat dementia. The first drug of this class prescribed for dementia was tacrine. This medication is now rarely used, as it gained a reputation for causing liver damage and intolerable side effects. Some, including Dr. William Summers, the man who was largely responsible for developing tacrine as a treatment for dementia, believe that tacrine's bad reputation is undeserved. In any case, the consensus has been that the more recently developed cholinesterase inhibitors, including Aricept, Razadyne (formerly called Reminyl), and Exelon, are better tolerated due to fewer side effects.

The cholinesterase inhibitors act primarily by blocking the breakdown of the neurotransmitter acetylcholine by the cholinesterase enzymes in the brain. This increases the amount of acetylcholine in the brain and leads to increase in the activation of nicotinic and muscarinic subtypes of acetylcholine receptors in brain tissue. As you might suspect, nicotinic receptors do indeed respond to the same nicotine that is found in tobacco. One good thing that smoking tobacco can do, among the many terrible things it does to the body, is to stimulate nicotinic receptors, which can improve clarity of thought. Unfortunately, the effects of nicotine wear off quickly, thus medicines such as cholinesterase inhibitors, whose effects are far more long lasting, are more beneficial. The name of the other acetylcholine receptor, the muscarinic receptor, comes from the name of the poisonous, hallucinogenic mushroom *Amanita muscaria*. This mushroom contains the substance muscarine, which potently blocks activity at muscarinic receptors in the brain. Antagonizing muscarinic receptors can cause hallucination and delirium. Many medications, often as a side effect, can block muscarinic receptors and produce similar effects. The diphenhydramine that is contained in many over-the-counter sleep aids is a potent muscarinic antagonist, which is why most doctors will strongly discourage its use in elderly people. Along with improving cognitive function, due to stimulation of nicotinic receptors, the cholinesterase inhibitors can also decrease confusion and hallucinations in patients with dementia by increasing activity at muscarinic receptors. This is why cholinesterase inhibitors are such an important treatment of not only Alzheimer's dementia, but also Lewy body dementia, a form of dementia in which visual hallucinations are prominent.

The cholinesterase inhibitors Aricept, Razadyne, and Exelon are quite similar in their effectiveness, although many believe that Razadyne offers a slight advantage due to extra ability to enhance activity at nicotinic receptors. I have used all three with success in different patients. The FDA has approved the use of these drugs for mild to moderate dementia, although many if not most physicians will start or continue the use of these medicines in patients with severe dementia as well. This is due to the fact that many patients will show improvements in behavior even if they exhibit no cognitive improvements, which makes the use of the medications still worthwhile. These drugs play an important role in the treatment of Lewy body dementia, regardless of severity.

The cholinesterase inhibitors are not approved for treatment of MCI, nor can they be prescribed for normal individuals hoping to avoid dementia. Nonetheless, there is data suggesting that adults with perfectly normal cognitive function could benefit from the use of these medications. A study published in the well-regarded professional journal *Neurology* in 2002 showed that thirty days of treatment with a low dose of Aricept improved the ability of licensed airplane pilots to perform complex tasks they had learned on a flight simulator. These pilots, who averaged fifty-two years of age, performed better than a matching group of pilots who underwent similar training without benefit of Aricept. There is also data showing that acetylcholine helps regulate the production and processing of amyloid precursor protein in the brain. Decreases in acetylcholine activity can cause accumulation of amyloid. Since this pathological process begins well before any cognitive dysfunction can be measured by standard tests, it stands to reason that drugs such as the cholinesterase inhibitors, or herbs and supplements that enhance acetylcholine activity, would be useful before dementia is diagnosed.

Memantine is a medication that has been in use in Germany for over twenty years to treat dementia and a variety of brain disorders, including Parkinson's disease, stroke, epilepsy, central nervous system trauma, amyotrophic lateral sclerosis (ALS), major depression, drug dependence, and chronic pain. The mechanism of action of memantine is fascinating. It acts primarily to antagonize, or block, activity at a receptor in the brain called the NMDA receptor. This action is interesting given the fact that many NMDA antagonists, including the so-called club drug ketamine and the infamous PCP, can have hallucinogenic, mind-altering effects. However, whereas those mind-altering drugs block all activity at the NMDA receptor, the mechanism of action of memantine allows it to block only abnormal stimulation of the NMDA receptor, while allowing physiologically normal activation of the receptor to proceed unimpeded. Thus, memantine can be thought of as reducing the "noise" of abnormal NMDA stimulation. It allows operation of the brain with less static and without stimulating hallucinations or other unwanted adverse effects. Memantine is also likely to offer some protection of neurons, as excess NMDA receptor activation can lead to toxic levels of calcium in the neuron, which in turn can lead to cell death.

In 2003, the FDA approved the sale of memantine in the United States for the treatment of moderate to severe Alzheimer's dementia. They have also allowed the combined treatment of memantine and a cholinesterase inhibitor for patients with severe dementia. Although memantine and cholinesterase inhibitors rarely do more than slow down the degenerative processes of dementia, there have actually been instances in which cognitive function was significantly improved for a number of weeks after starting the combined treatment. A number of clinical trials have shown that memantine can be helpful in earlier, milder stages of Alzheimer's, and it has been prescribed in Germany and other countries for this purpose. However, whereas the FDA has approved the use of the cholinesterase inhibitors for mild to moderate stages of Alzheimer's dementia, it has so far rejected the use of memantine for those earlier stages of the illness.

PRESCRIPTION MEDICATIONS WITH PROMISING EFFECTS

Several prescription medications may help reduce the risk of dementia despite being approved by the FDA as treatments for other conditions. It has been recognized for a number of years that the class of drugs known as statins, which are used to lower cholesterol in the blood, may also decrease the risk of dementia. Because high LDL cholesterol increases the risk of cardiovascular disease, which in turn increases the risk of dementia, these findings were not terribly surprising. About 25 percent of the cholesterol in the body can be found in the brain. Cholesterol is so important to the brain that it does not depend on cholesterol in the blood for its supply. The brain makes its own. There is evidence that increasing the cholesterol burden inside the brain can increase the rate of production of amyloid protein, which in turn exacerbates the deposition of amyloid into the destructive plaques. Studies have shown that statins can reduce the synthesis of cholesterol inside the brain as well as deposition of beta amyloid protein in brain tissue. Thus, beneficial effects of statins could be due in part to decreasing the production of cholesterol in the brain.

Curiously, a study published in one of the most highly regarded medical journals in the world, *The Lancet*, revealed that statins offered protection from dementia to people regardless of whether they had high or normal cholesterol. Moreover, not all medications that reduce serum cholesterol also reduce the risk of developing dementia. Thus it seems likely that the statins also help prevent dementia through mechanisms that have little or nothing to do with cholesterol. Several different statin drugs have been found to decrease inflammatory responses and oxidative stress in brain. They may also increase brain concentrations of BDNF, which is involved in stimulating nerve growth and neurogenesis. I am obliged to note that, overall, studies using statins to prevent dementia have been rather disappointing. However, this may reflect the complexity of dementia and the fact that many factors play a role in its initiation and progression.

An important caveat in regard to treatment with statins is that this class of medicines inhibits not only the synthesis of cholesterol, but also of the critical substance co-enzyme Q10. Thus, anyone taking a statin should supplement with CoQ10. I discuss this substance and its importance, as well as how to supplement the diet with it, in chapter 6.

Medicines that are beginning to be seen as possibly playing a role in preventing Alzheimer's dementia in people with diabetes type 2 include the glitazones. Glitazones are oral hypoglycemic medications that include rosiglitazone (Avandia) and pioglitazone (Actos). These medicines improve the body's response to insulin, but they appear to have many other benefits that are related to improving insulin sensitivity. They act primarily by stimulating a substance called PPAR in cells of the body. In the brain, PPAR stimulation not only enhances the action of insulin, but also stimulates disposal of amyloid and decreases the intensity of inflammatory processes that occur when amyloid begins to form plaques in brain tissue. An encouraging, but not fully replicated, finding has been that treatment with rosiglitazone helps preserve cognitive function in patients with early Alzheimer's dementia. As with all medicines, the glitazones have the potential to cause harm in some people. Glitazones are medications that have recently come under scrutiny by the FDA for possibly increasing the risk of heart failure and death from heart disease. The possible adverse effects of glitazones remain a controversial subject in the field of medicine, and they are certainly not medications to be taken for frivolous reasons. Nonetheless, if you or a loved one have both diabetes type 2 and other risk factors for developing dementia, a discussion with a physician would be worthwhile.

Another promising treatment for dementia is a medication already in use for a different purpose. A class of medications known as angiotensin receptor blockers, or ARBs, are used to treat high blood pressure in patients who have not responded well to more traditional, and less expensive, medications. High blood pressure itself is a risk factor for Alzheimer's and vascular dementia, and almost any kind of treatment reduces that risk. However, recent studies have found ARBs to have an unexpectedly powerful ability to prevent the progression of neurodegeneration, and this may reflect effects beyond the mere reduction of blood pressure. A recent study at the Boston University School of Medicine found, over a five-year period, that patients treated with ARBs for high blood pressure were 40 percent less likely to develop dementia than patients treated with other medications for blood pressure. It also appeared to slow the progression of symptoms in patients who were eventually diagnosed with dementia.

Angiotensin is a natural substance in the body that acts in various ways to increase blood pressure.[1] It is also found in the brain, where it has long been known to play an important role in controlling fluid intake and thirst in mammals, including humans. An impressive demonstration in neurophysiology laboratories is to inject angiotensin directly into the brain of a rat, which will then immediately stop what it is doing and run off to get a drink of water. Angiotensin is produced in the body through the action of an enzyme called angiotensin converting enzyme, or ACE, and medications known as ACE inhibitors, which block this enzyme, are an important and effective class of medications for treating high blood pressure. As is often the case, angiotensin may have other, hitherto unexplored effects on the brain. Although the significance of the findings remains to be determined, studies have found that ACE and angiotensin are overactive in some animal models of Alzheimer's dementia. It is puzzling why ARBs, which block the effects of angiotensin in the brain, would be so much more effective in slowing neurodegeneration than ACE inhibitors, which block the production of angiotensin in the brain and rest of the body. It is possible that different subtypes of angiotensin receptors have different effects on brain activity, and that these receptors are differentially affected by the ARBs. In any case, such powerful results from a class of medication already found to be relatively safe for human patients is good news.

It has long been known that many medications in the class known as non-steroidal anti-inflammatory drugs, or NSAIDs, can reduce the risk of developing Alzheimer's dementia and possibly other forms of dementia, including Lewy body. Some of these medications, including ibuprofen, naproxen, orudis, and aspirin, have long been available as over-the-counter medications. The NSAID about which there is the most data to show ability to reduce the risk of dementia is ibuprofen. This beneficial effect of ibuprofen has been found from observing a reduction in the frequency of Alzheimer's dementia among people who have taken ibuprofen daily for many years as treatment for arthritis and other painful inflammatory conditions.

The NSAIDs might act by a number of different mechanisms to prevent or slow down the neurodegenerative processes of Alzheimer's and other forms of dementia. They decrease inflammation, reduce production of amyloid, decrease hyperphosphorylation of tau protein, and help prevent

---

1. When I taught neuropharmacology in university classes, a line that could always be relied upon to evoke eye rolls and a chorus of groans was my assertion that, contrary to popular belief, Angie O'Tensin is *not* a famous Irish folksinger.

the addition of sugars to proteins that end in the production of advanced glycation endproducts that ramp up the inflammation processes in the brain. They appear to be extraordinarily useful medications. There are several NSAIDs available by prescription only, such as flurbiprofen, that more readily cross the blood-brain barrier than the over-the-counter varieties, and thus are more effective in producing beneficial effects in the brain. A recent study published in *Lancet Neurology* found that daily administration of atrenflurbil, a special form of flurbiprofen, slowed the rate of cognitive decline in patients already diagnosed with mild Alzheimer's dementia. Medications with benefits for such individuals are rare and noteworthy.

Ibuprofen and other NSAIDs are available without prescription at any pharmacy or convenience store, but the potential for these medicines to cause serious harm should not be underestimated. They can cause significant ulceration and bleeding problems in the stomach, and they are related in their actions to the COX-2 inhibitors that have become infamous for increasing the risk of cardiac death. Before starting daily use of any NSAID, it is important to discuss the plan with your doctor.

MEDICINES IN THE PIPELINE

A very interesting medication being studied for the treatment of Alzheimer's dementia is Dimebon. Dimebon was first developed in Russia as an antihistamine to treat the symptoms of allergy. It seems to have been found quite by accident that the drug had dramatic effects on the cognitive function of patients diagnosed with Alzheimer's dementia. One of the first studies of the effects of Dimebon, performed at the Moscow Center of Gerontology, found that after eight weeks of therapy with the medication, the cognitive functions and mood of Alzheimer's patients were substantially improved without ill effects.

Although Dimebon was developed as an antihistamine, it is very unlikely that this aspect of its action is responsible for its effects on cognitive function. In fact, further study has determined that Dimebon also produces effects quite similar to those of the two types of medications that are currently FDA-approved to treat dementia. Dimebon acts to increase acetylcholine activity by blocking its destruction by the enzymes acetylcholinesterase and butyrylcholinesterase. Moreover, Dimebon appears to block abnormal activation of the NMDA receptor in the brain, in much the same manner as the anti-dementia medication memantine. Dimebon, like tacrine, a drug approved for treatment of dementia that has fallen into disfavor in the United

States, has also been found to block some of the toxic effects of amyloid on mitochondria, which are the energy powerhouses in every cell of the body, including the brain.

Extra benefits of Dimebon, particularly its ability to improve mood in patients with dementia, are likely due to its antidepressant-like effects of blocking the monoamine oxidase enzymes that destroy the neurotransmitters serotonin, norepinephrine, and dopamine in the brain. Dimebon also enhances activity at a receptor in the brain called the AMPA subtype of glutamate receptors. This is a characteristic common among antidepressant medications. The FDA has now approved large-scale clinical studies of the use of Dimebon in the treatment of dementia. Hopefully, we will soon be able to determine if it lives up to its promise as a treatment that can actually help improve cognitive function to a significant degree, rather than simply slow down the decline in function as current treatments tend to do.

There are a number of other medications in the research pipeline that will be coming available over the next few years. These include medications such as secretase inhibitors that prevent the splitting of APP into the sticky, dangerous form of amyloid, and even vaccines that stimulate immune cells in the brain to attack and rid its tissues of the abnormal amyloid proteins. A medication with the ungainly name of "bapineuzumab" acts by the mechanism of passive immunization to amyloid. That is, it is an antibody to amyloid that is similar in many ways to the final product the immune cells in the body would produce. In this way, antibodies that attack the amyloid protein deposits can be obtained while bypassing the body's own natural immune system response. In several human subjects, stimulating a strong natural immune response against amyloid in the brain has proved to be dangerous.

One of the most remarkable reports of effects of medication in Alzheimer's dementia has been the finding that injection of the TNF antagonist etanercept directly into the cerebrospinal fluid that bathes the brain produces a dramatic and rapid reversal of some of the cognitive deficits of Alzheimer's dementia. A promising medication, tramiprosate, crosses the so-called blood-brain barrier, from the bloodstream into the brain, and binds to amyloid before it is able to crystallize on existing deposits of amyloid. This allows the brain to dispose of the amyloid and stop enlargement of plaques.

Another unique and promising treatment for Alzheimer's dementia is NAP. NAP is a short fragment of a natural brain protein called activity-dependent neuroprotective protein. NAP protects brain cells against a number of different insults, and recent tests are suggesting that it may improve function in patients with dementia. NAP appears to interact with tau protein, which is the protein that in abnormal conditions accumulates as neurofibrillary tangles in the brain of patients with Alzheimer's dementia. In a recent preliminary study, NAP administered as a nasal spray twice a day improved the cognitive function of patients with MCI. Whereas many drugs in development are directed toward reducing the burden of beta amyloid plaques in the brain, NAP appears to be the first medication that acts by reducing neurofibrillary tangles of tau protein in brain tissue. Since it acts by a very different mechanism, it might be possible to add NAP to treatments directed at amyloid accumulation to obtain even better results. It is also encouraging that NAP appears to work in individuals with MCI. It would be preferable to treat people in the earliest stages of cognitive loss rather than simply trying to prevent further loss after people are already suffering disabling forms of dementia.

An old and well-known substance, methylene blue, has been found to enhance learning in rats.[2] It was thought that it enhanced cognitive function by increasing metabolic rates of mitochondria in the brain. Recently, however, it has been found that methylene blue is yet another substance that can reduce accumulation of neurofibrillary tangles of tau protein in brain tissue. A preliminary study in England has now shown that methylene blue, referred to by the name Rember, can slow and virtually stop the decline in cognitive function seen in patients with Alzheimer's dementia. In the relatively small study, in which 321 patients took part, those who received methylene blue had a more than 80 percent reduction in loss of cognitive function when compared to those who did not receive the drug. In some patients, no decline in cognitive function was noted over the nineteen months of the study. Thus methylene blue joins NAP as a treatment that may soon be available to reverse some of the cognitive losses of Alzheimer's dementia by ridding the brain of neurofibrillary tangles.

---

2. An old prank popular in fraternities with a high percentage of nerdy science majors was to slip methylene blue into a brother's cola and wait for him to shriek with horror when upon his next trip to the bathroom he finds that his urine has turned blue.

9

THE DEMENTIA EPIDEMIC AND HOW TO AVOID IT

In a Nutshell

WHAT IS DEMENTIA?

- The definition of dementia, according to the American Psychiatric Association's *Diagnostic and Statistical Manual IV* is: A condition of loss of memory, accompanied by impairment of decision-making or personality change. These changes must be severe enough to impair an individual's work, social activities, or relationships with others.
- When memory disturbances are present, but they do not significantly affect a person's work, social activities, or relationships, the condition is referred to as mild cognitive impairment, or MCI.
- Alzheimer's dementia is the most common and well-known dementia. However, it accounts for only about half of cases of dementia. Other forms of dementia include vascular, Lewy body, and frontotemporal dementias.
- The diagnosis of dementia can be made only after other medical and psychiatric diagnoses have been ruled out. Thus, evaluation of changes in cognitive function must include a good physical examination, blood tests, and consideration of psychiatric contribution.
- Some psychiatric conditions, such as major depression, and some medical conditions, such as low thyroid hormone, vitamin deficiencies, and sleep apnea, can mimic dementia. If diagnosed and treated

promptly, loss of cognitive function due to these problems can sometimes be reversed.

THE CAUSES OF DEMENTIA

- Although some people are genetically predisposed to one or another
  form of dementia, in most cases dementia is due to poor lifestyle
  choices. For most people, dementia is avoidable.
- Studies have shown that individuals who immigrate to developed countries, depart from the ways of their traditional cultures, and adopt the
  lifestyles of the modern societies are at increased risk for dementia.
- In the majority of cases, genes are neither necessary nor sufficient to
  cause dementia. Genes we inherit from our parents merely tend to
  determine the primary ways in which bad diet, stress, and the other
  unhealthy aspects of lifestyle will affect the brain and cognitive function.
- Metabolic syndrome is a major risk factor for all types of dementia.
- Metabolic syndrome is a risk factor for heart disease and diabetes,
  which themselves are risk factors for dementia.
- Metabolic syndrome is diagnosed by the presence of high blood pressure, high fasting blood glucose, high triglycerides, low HDL (the
  good cholesterol), and abdominal obesity.
- The underlying cause of metabolic syndrome is insulin resistance.
- Metabolic syndrome is often the result of too much sugar, too much
  saturated fat, too much stress, too little sleep, not enough exercise, and
  bad health habits.
- Other risk factors for dementia are major depression, sleep apnea,
  poor educational background, boring work, overindulgence in smoking
  and drinking, head injury, poor dental care, social isolation, inflammatory processes, hormone imbalances, environmental toxins, and a
  growing list of bacteria and viruses.

HOW TO AVOID DEMENTIA

- To stay free of dementia you must fight metabolic syndrome, diabetes,
  heart disease, and other physical risk factors through diet, prudent
  supplementation, weight loss, exercise, good sleep, and stress reduction.

- For most people, the diet that best reduces the risk of metabolic syndrome, heart disease, diabetes, and dementia is the Mediterranean diet.
- The key features of the Mediterranean diet are fruits and vegetables high in fiber, less red meat and more deep sea fish, less butter and more olive oil, garlic, red wine, spices rich in antioxidants, and few sweets.
- The best diet for weight loss may not be the Mediterranean diet. For most people, high protein and good fat tend to cut appetite and make weight loss easier.
- Diet plus exercise is the surest way to lose weight.
- Ideal weight for men is 106 pounds for the first 5 feet, then 6 pounds for each additional inch of height. For women, this weight is 100 pounds for the first 5 feet, then 5 pounds for each additional inch of height. Add 10 extra pounds for being over fifty years old, and add or subtract 10 pounds for having a large or small frame.
- There are many herbs, vitamins, and nutraceuticals that can be taken as supplements to help avoid or delay the progression of dementia.
- The actions to look for in a useful combination of supplements include: antioxidant effects, anti-inflammatory effects, enhancement of acetylcholine, stimulation of neuron growth, anti-amyloid effects, and prevention of metabolic syndrome.
- Steer clear of environmental toxins by drinking clean water, breathing clean air, and eating fresh, uncontaminated food.
- In some cases, medications are necessary to avoid metabolic syndrome and its adverse effects.
- Medications may be needed to improve cognitive function and prevent further decline in the early stages of dementia. Currently, the FDA-approved medications include the NMDA receptor antagonist memantine (Namenda) and the cholinesterase inhibitors Aricept, Razadyne, and Exelon.
- Do not despair; research is ongoing, and there are many new medications on the horizon.
- To avoid dementia you must exercise your mind as well as your body. You must keep learning throughout life and strengthen your mind with challenging work and interesting pastimes.
- Use books, puzzles, and games as supplements, not replacements, for doing intellectually stimulating things with interesting people.
- A good marriage, where the spouse is also a friend and confidant, is the best of all possibilities.

- People who are able to maintain close friendships through adulthood and old age are less likely to develop dementia.
- People can and should continue to develop and grow emotionally and spiritually through adulthood and old age. Those who do not are at higher risk for dementia.
- Learn to love unconditionally, fulfill your dreams, find meaning and contentment, forgive, and come to peace with yourself.

INDEX